The Resilience Blueprint

The Resilience Blueprint

Find your resilience type.
Beat burnout.
Bounce back better.

Dr Dani Gordon

First published in Great Britain in 2023 by Orion Spring,
an imprint of The Orion Publishing Group Ltd
Carmelite House, 50 Victoria Embankment
London EC4Y 0DZ

An Hachette UK Company

1 3 5 7 9 10 8 6 4 2

A CIP catalogue record for this book is
available from the British Library.

ISBN (Trade Paperback) 978 1 4091 9708 9
ISBN (eBook) 978 1 4091 9710 2
ISBN (Audio) 978 1 3987 0004 8

Typeset by Born Group
Printed in Great Britain by Clays Ltd, Elcograf S.p.A.

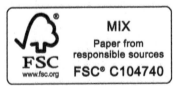

FSC
www.fsc.org

MIX
Paper from
responsible sources
FSC® C104740

www.orionbooks.co.uk

To my son River, my greatest
joy and resilience teacher

CONTENTS

WHAT IS RESILIENCE?

Meg came to see me in the clinic for a number of health concerns that, on the surface, seemed unrelated. She felt tired but on edge. Small stresses had started to feel bigger lately and she felt a general sense of 'overwhelm' most days. She had always been, as she put it, Type A, but things had definitely got worse over the last few years. She had started to have palpitations and had trouble getting to sleep at night. The confusing part for Meg was that she did everything 'right.' She went to ashtanga yoga three times a week, ate organic food, drank plenty of water and took a mountain of supplements each morning. She tried to be mindful. She didn't smoke or binge drink and she did 10,000 steps most days. How was it possible to still feel stressed out and overwhelmed, living what was surely a 'super-healthy lifestyle'? As she said to me at the time, 'What is the point of doing all this healthy stuff if I still don't feel amazing or even OK many days? Wasn't the whole point of living "healthy" to make me feel better and more "resilient", as everyone is always going on about?'

If Meg's story seems relatable, you are not alone. In fact, this experience of the mismatch between an apparently super-healthy lifestyle and a lack of translation into feeling awesome is extremely common. Luckily, it doesn't have to be this way. You can end this confusing and frustrating cycle, to feel happier, healthier and more fulfilled, without a crazy wellness regimen or drinking nothing but celery juice. The secret to becoming more resilient is not trying to live a picture-perfect life, doing more exercise classes or swearing off anything slightly unhealthy for ever. I have found, working with countless patients, that they tend to break down into four distinct resilience 'types', and each of these needs a very different approach to find balance, energy and the ability to deal with life's ups and downs. Once you know your type, which we'll explore in Chapter One, you can focus your energies in the right way and avoid the specific pitfalls that could be holding you back from truly thriving in hectic modern life.

For example, depending on your resilience type, a super-strong ashtanga yoga practice may be great for your physique but the exact opposite of the type of mind–body practice you may need to balance your brain and mind. Instead, you might just need to rekindle some joy in your life or take back control of your energy levels. The resilience blueprint presented in this book is about finding the bespoke approach that fits you, and no one else.

Back at my clinic, Meg and I worked together to create a plan to help lower her stress load, get her sleeping well again and decrease her anxiety symptoms during the day – and we did it by actually simplifying all the wellness things she was doing. It turned out that some of her supplements contained stimulating ingredients that were probably making her feel more on edge (like green tea extract and panax ginseng). We cut her supplements right down, focusing on the few that really did make a difference and added some CBD oil. Meg swapped one of her high-intensity yoga sessions for a restorative gentle yoga class to help her wind down better. I gave her a super-simple breathing practice to use for a few minutes each day at her desk at work and in the evenings. We made more space in her day and evenings for 'doing nothing' and gave her the permission to make this a priority instead of tightly scheduling every minute of the day. We focused on simple-to-make, nourishing foods with healthy fats rather than the low-fat diet she had been following. And we got rid of caffeine for a while, but swapped it for an herbal tea latte that helps balance stress hormones and keep energy going without the crashes. In three months, Meg was feeling calmer, more confident and less edgy.

Until recently, 'resilience' was a bit of a vague concept in the medical world. Despite overall agreement that it is essential to be physically and mentally resilient to life's demands, there has been very little medical consensus on how to measure resilience. There is no blood test, no single resilience gene and no single pill that will make you instantly more resilient. This is one reason why most doctors can usually offer little guidance when you are essentially well but not feeling your best.

For many people, when they hear the word 'resilience', the first thing that comes to mind is mental toughness, grit, 'pushing through' and 'trying harder'. However, as a doctor, I believe this is not really what resilience is all about. I prefer to define resilience as the ability to 'bounce back', from inevitable life setbacks, stresses and difficulties and even 'bounce forward' to feeling better than before. True resilience is about how we can maintain the best quality of life and sense of wellbeing as we go through life's ups and downs. Resilience doesn't mean leading a life of purity and zen-like calm – that's impossible anyway. It's about meeting yourself where you are and being adaptable and capable. I want to reassure you that you can be resilient at any stage of life and no matter what health challenges you may be living with. That is because the core of resilience is the ability to keep adapting and adjusting your whole being in the face of significant adversity or challenging life circumstances. It's also about being kinder and gentler to yourself rather than pushing harder or going faster through life. One of the most resilient people I know has recovered twice from stage 4 cancer and although it is highly unlikely she is 'cured' permanently, she lives each day in a state of what most definitely is high resilience.

Some people may be more naturally skilled at being resilient in specific areas of life than others – think of someone who never catches colds or flu, for example, but often experiences crippling overwhelm. But thankfully we are not stuck with the resilience level we have right now. The way I like to define resilience is as a dynamic state of balance in the brain and in the body. Being truly and sustainably resilient is a dance between stress that can become toxic and the protective factors that keep it in check. It's about holistic health.

Resilience is also a set of skills that can be trained, enhanced and shifted. This is true even if you feel you have lived in a state of low resilience for many years, or possibly your entire life. In essence, this book is here to demonstrate how resilience is not something you either have or you don't – it can always be learned and improved upon.

Another counter-intuitive thing about resilience is that to build it and grow it, we actually need to experience setbacks and adversities. No one ever built resilience living a perfectly easeful life. You can think of resilience as a muscle you have to flex to make it stronger, just like going to the gym and doing those horrible planks to get stronger abs. Even traumatic events in our lives can be a doorway to resilience, a discovery I have made through personal experience and in treating many thousands of patients in my integrative holistic medicine practice over the past decade. In challenging circumstances it can help to know that having negative experiences does not doom us, but instead they are crucial to our resilience journey. Setbacks of all kinds can lead to higher levels of mental wellbeing, functioning and gratitude on a brain level if we can integrate them successfully. This is quite comforting since setbacks, traumas and negative life events are pretty much impossible to avoid.

Resilience is also not a you-have-it-or-you-don't, all-or-nothing sort of thing; it's a continually evolving state of being. Some people may be more naturally emotionally resilient and find it easy to stay positive when the going gets tough, while others may be more physically resilient in certain ways, like my mother-in-law who has an immune system of steel: when the rest of the family had all the symptoms of Covid in the spring of 2020, she had barely more than a day's sniffle. We all have our unique strengths and unique set of challenges and, as you will soon discover, our own resilience type. How resilient we feel also changes over time. It waxes and wanes with the ups and downs of life (which is totally normal).

So now that you know resilience is about your bounce-back factor, how do we actually go about hacking it, breaking it down and finding out what it's all about? The science of resilience is also becoming a new field in medicine, and one that I have spent over a decade studying and using to treat patients and help them on their healing journeys. When people ask what sort of medicine I practise, I used to have a long, convoluted answer since, as an integrative medicine specialist, I integrate things that on the surface may seem totally unrelated. Along my journey I've studied things as diverse as traditional yogic meditation and breathing in a remote Indian ashram, high-tech brain biofeedback and brainwave scanning and the therapeutic use of psychedelics and medical cannabis. All of these experiences, expertise areas and tools had one thing in common: they were all tools I used to help my patients become more resilient. This was regardless of whether the patient suffered from anxiety and stress or a serious chronic illness that had no cure. It is the integrative holistic application of these practices in a systematic way that has made the big difference to my patients, rather than a single 'quick fix'.

I've also been applying resilience as medicine to my own life to help reduce my stress levels, look and feel more vitalized (and yes, youthful too) and, most importantly, become happier and more fulfilled in hectic modern life without having to retreat to a meditation cave for ever. Resilience is truly the science of integration – you don't have to retreat from life to become resilient, you just need to adapt.

But don't worry, building your resilience doesn't have to be complicated, or take a huge amount of time. Once you have defined your resilience type, you can start with simple small changes each day to start tapping into your bounce-back superpowers. Learning more about your own resilience type will help you understand why you may have been frustrated with previous failed attempts to build your ability to roll with life's punches.

I believe there are three core principles of resilience as medicine:

1. We can change our brains and bodies no matter where we are starting from. No one is too old, too tired or too sick to become more resilient. We can start wherever we are.
2. The integration of many factors is key to resilience. Let go of the idea of the magic bullet or the quick fix. Some of the core

elements to integrate include what we eat and what supplements we take, how we think, how we relax and let go, how we recover from traumas, how we enjoy life, how we move our bodies, and our environment – both internal and external.

3. Knowing your resilience type will help you cut through the confusing world of wellbeing, with its often contradictory messages.

The goal of *The Resilience Blueprint* is to help optimize your bounce-back factor, not just so you can be healthier, but so that you can become the best possible version of yourself. Upping your resilience game will help you truly live life to the fullest no matter what might be going on for you and those around you.

In Part One, I will introduce you to all the different aspects of resilience, and you will discover your resilience type with a simple quiz. You will learn about where you sit on my Resilience Spectrum (and this will change throughout your life). I will also teach you what factors in our genes, our brains, our cells, our food, our thoughts and our environment contribute to our resilience level and the top ten resilience temperament traits we can all learn.

After you get your resilience score and find out your personal resilience type, I will teach you how to make your brain, mind and body more resilient, depending on your natural strengths, gifts and challenges. Knowing your type will also give you a starting point to work from on your resilience journey. This means going from 'stress victim' and/or 'the burnout zone' to becoming a resilience rock star who can live more of your life in what I like to call our 'thrive zone'.

In Part Two, we will dive into my resilience toolkit, including the optimal diet, supplements, mind–body practices and other tools for healing and building a more resilient you. We will explore how some of these practices and 'resilience hacks' can be incorporated into a busy lifestyle to reduce stress and burnout in each type.

Part Three will give you an eight-week resilience plan you can follow, with instructions on how to tweak it for your type.

By reading this far, you have already taken the first and hardest step towards resilience! The best time to start making a small shift is always the present moment.

I hope in these pages you will find the tools and confidence to start or deepen your resilience journey, no matter where you are starting from. Resilience is a lifelong journey of growth. So if you are already feeling quite bouncy, amazing! This book and the eight-week plan will help you reach new heights of mental and physical performance and wellbeing. If, however, you are reading this from a low, vulnerable place and feel like you have tried everything and almost given up, I hope this will be the start of a new chapter in your life, giving you hope and confidence that things can get better no matter what life has thrown at you so far.

Wherever you are now, the number one rule is to remember to be kind and patient to yourself and approach this new journey with curiosity and patience. My advice to you is that this seemingly small mental practice alone will set you on the path to a more resilient, happy and thriving version of you.

PART ONE

How Resilient Are You?

CHAPTER ONE

FINDING YOUR RESILIENCE TYPE

As an integrative medicine doctor I have so many tools at my disposal, everything from nutritional medicine to high-tech brain scans. But without doubt one of the most useful tools I have found is helping my patients identify their resilience type. Without knowing this key piece of information about how your brain and your body function, you can keep making the same 'resilience mistakes' and, despite putting in massive effort, you may struggle to enter your thrive zone.

I developed a system to help assess how resilient you are right now at this stage of your life, and to help you find your 'resilience type'. It's important to note that it is possible to be a mix of types, and in fact many people will identify as a mix of two types. And your resilience type may change with your circumstances, so it is worth checking in with yourself regularly to assess how you might be feeling.

I define the four resilience types as:

- **Wound-up warriors**
  Naturally high strung, these people have a hard time coming back to a calm baseline in the nervous system, brain and body and avoiding chronic hyperarousal. They often identify as being 'high-stress' people. However, they can be highly effective and are the go-to people for getting the job done.

- **Moody warriors**
  Their biggest challenge is maintaining a positive healthy mood balance, Finding the joy in day-to-day life can be a challenge too. However, when they are in balance, they are often the life and soul of a party.

- **Exhausted warriors**
  They tend to burn themselves out more than other types, using more energy than they have in the tank and feeling totally drained. Their challenge is managing and supporting energy levels on a brain, body and cellular level. They often identify as being less energetic than average and need more sleep too. On the upside, exhausted warriors tend to be highly intuitive and empathetic.

- **Scattered warriors**
  These people get distracted easily and can find it hard to focus, although they have a constant stream of new ideas. Memory is not their strong suit, from remembering where they put things to dates in the calendar. Maintaining mental focus and clarity to support optimal thinking and concentration is their challenge. They often say they feel a bit 'ADD' even if they have never been formally diagnosed with attention deficit disorder or ADHD. They tend to be highly creative in some way and are great innovators.

As you can see, each type comes with hidden superpowers too, not just weaknesses.

If you have been struggling for many years in multiple areas of your life, these types can get a bit jumbled up and you may feel like all of them sound like you! However, by taking the quiz, you can see which type fits where you are now, to get a reference for where to start. This is extra important if you are struggling, because reducing overwhelm is key to starting on your resilience journey. That is because overwhelm tends to make us freeze up and avoid taking any action at all.

Other people may also find they are more of an even balance and in different areas of their life one resilience type emerges more strongly than the rest. For example, at work you may find you have more wound-up warrior tendencies while your primary type may be scattered warrior. However, most people do find they are at least slightly more dominant in one type overall and that is the one to work with first.

Now we will take the Resilience Type quiz so you know where to start with your resilience journey. Again, if you are a combination of two types, this assessment will help you choose which one to start with.

Once you know your type, I'll explain about each in much more detail.

Resilience Type Quiz

SCALE

Mark each answer with a number as follows:
3 = not me at all/never
2 = a bit like me/sometimes
1 = like me/often
0 = very much like me/very often

SECTION A

- I get physical body sensations such as heart palpitations/racing heartbeat, chest tightness, sweating or feeling like I can't catch my breath when I'm not exercising.
- I grind my teeth at night and/or have jaw tension.
- I have physical muscle tension in my body such as neck, back-aches and chronic muscle tension that is hard to get rid of.
- I experience a sense of 'overwhelm'.
- I have trouble falling asleep easily.
- I have gut symptoms (e.g. bloating, gas, pain, diarrhoea or

constipation) that tend to get worse with stress or emotional upset despite conventional medical tests coming back as 'normal'.
- I have to rely on sleeping medications or supplements to get to sleep and/or stay asleep.
- I have trouble shutting off my thoughts, especially before bed, even when I try to relax.
- I get headaches.
- I am sensitive to loud or sudden noises and tend to be 'jumpy' if someone or something surprises me.
- Caffeine makes me feel jittery especially if I have too much.
- I find it hard to meditate.
- I have a hard time 'doing nothing'.
- I tend to be a worrier.
- I feel 'stressed out'.

SECTION B

- I feel more tired after I exercise.
- I experience brain fog.
- I get mentally fatigued easily.
- I get afternoon energy crashes.
- I need caffeine in the morning to feel 'normal'.
- I feel like I need three-day weekends to recover after the work week.
- I have less desire for sex or a lower libido than I used to.*
- I wake up feeling tired a lot even after eight hours of sleep.
- I need at least nine hours of sleep to feel optimally rested.
- I get sick often and it takes me longer to recover from colds and flus than average.
- I have low thyroid or borderline-normal thyroid issues.
- I have experienced burnout in the past or am currently on the exhaustion end of burning out.

---

* low libido can be caused by a number of issues, so if you scored a 0 or 1 for this question, consider speaking to your health practitioner about hormone function testing to ensure there are no issues with hormonal imbalances such as low testosterone or other issues.

- It takes me one week to fully recover from a 'night out' when I went to bed very late.
- I get bad hangovers lasting more than twenty-four hours when I drink alcohol even in moderation.
- I tend to put others' needs before my own.

SECTION C

- I find I am easily irritated by small problems or things that build up.
- I experience low moods for 'no reason'.
- I have negative self-talk or repeated negative thinking that is hard to stop or 'break the loop'.
- I have difficulty controlling my emotions or tend to get mood swings.
- I tend to feel guilty.
- I have difficulty waking up in the morning without loud alarms.
- I have trouble motivating myself to exercise or go to a gym/yoga class, even though I try to psych myself up for it.
- I have found relaxation practices don't help me feel better or they make me feel more irritable.
- I experience a vague sense of mental suffering without knowing why.
- I have decreased desire for socializing and doing things I previously enjoyed.
- Feeling/finding happiness each day is a challenge.
- I feel a lack of purpose and meaning/fulfilment in daily life.
- Depression or other mood conditions run in my family.
- Alcohol is a tool I use to help unwind and feel good, especially after a stressful day.
- Without the aid of substances (including alcohol), I find it is hard for me to enjoy socializing or feel happy.

SECTION D

- I have noticed a decrease in my memory or misplace Items more than I used to.

- I find it hard to stick to a routine.
- I find it hard to plan in advance.
- I have problems focusing/concentrating, especially for prolonged periods of time.
- I have problems with filtering important from unimportant details in stories, conversations and work projects.
- I tend to procrastinate.
- I tend to rush to finish things
- I tend to get stressed around decision making and then not make any decision.
- I tend to daydream a lot, even when I am supposed to be focusing.
- I find it hard to stay organized, especially for long periods of time.
- I get bored easily.
- I thrive on high-stimulation sports and hobbies.
- I get hooked easily on social media apps, video games and other screen-based activities and find it hard to stop using them.
- I start multiple projects at the same time but sometimes have difficulty finishing them.
- I have been diagnosed with ADD/ADHD in the past as a child or more recently as an adult, *or* I strongly suspect I have it even though I don't have a formal diagnosis.

SCORING YOUR RESILIENCE MATRIX: GETTING YOUR TYPE

Add Up Your Total Score for A, B, C and D

A =

B =

C =

D =

Lowest Number = Your primary Resilience Type

The Four Resilience Types in Detail

Wound-up Warriors

If this is your resilience type, your main challenge is being able to return to a calm, cool and collected nervous-system 'baseline.' You may find you live a lot of your life in a state of hyperarousal or 'jacked-up' on stress 24/7. Balancing your wound-up or high-strung nature is key to feeling less anxiety and overwhelm, 'shutting off' thoughts easily, healing poor sleep and being able to get yourself into a calm, relaxed state 'on demand' in real life, which is your resilience key.

At first you may say, 'No, this is not me, the quiz is wrong, I don't "feel stressed" at all – I'm totally fine!' That is a very common response for this resilience type because often the stressed, jacked-up state has been there for so long that the nervous system and brain has learned to block it out. This is a brain-coping mechanism so that you don't totally crumble and can still function, but the downside is that you learn to live in a state of chronic stress and neurological 'wind-up'.

A typical initial reaction when I tell a new patient or client that this is their main type is to say, 'But I'm so relaxed/laid back, that just doesn't sound like me!' However, on further questioning, they come to accept that they are actually quite 'wound up', without being consciously aware of it. Because of the tendency towards perfectionism, many people who fall into this type are able to camouflage this 'wound-up' nature to all but those closest to them. The chronic 'wound-up' nature contributes to what I like to think of as brain and mind 'noise' turning the volume up over time until it starts to make things hard to hear or to think clearly. For example, 'body noise' can show up as physical sensations of stress and anxiety like shortness of breath and panic attacks as well as digestion issues. 'Mind noise' can show up as the inability to turn off mental chatter at times when you are trying to relax or, most classically, while you are trying to get to sleep. Often that chatter is repetitive loops rehashing something that happened that day or rehearsing for something you have to do tomorrow, or rethinking something you did or said.

This resilience type typically feels that they don't have time for things like meditating (boring!) or 'sitting and doing nothing'. They are always on the go and find it hard to find time to rest and rejuvenate. A holiday spent sitting on the beach on a sun lounger, curled up with a book, often sounds more like torture than heaven to a wound-up warrior. This predisposition to being tightly wound creates a brain and nervous system that is more reactive to small daily stresses and remains a bit 'on edge', waiting for the next stress to come along. Over time, the brain loses its ability to dial down the arousal levels in the brain and mind, even at times when you feel you are 'chilling out'.

When I ask these clients how their 'off switch' works, they often say, 'What off switch?' They have often never or very rarely experienced a state of true, peaceful calm unless they are totally exhausted and crashing into sleep.

The types of traits that lead to having no off switch are not necessarily 'bad', but like any trait, it can be a strength as well as a weakness depending on how it's managed. For example, being a high achiever who is always on the go can be very good for professional success, and often this resilience type excels professionally and can be found in positions of leadership. However, if this lack of switching off gets out of hand, the wound-up nature can lead to clinical anxiety disorder, toxic stress and burnout.

The good news is that once you are aware this is your type, you can turn your 'wound-up' nature into a superpower to achieve incredible things and lead a fulfilling life without the anxiety and toxic stress. You will learn to dial down your always-on nature and slow down. This is a skill I have had to learn over many years myself. I always tell people when they ask me why I do a consistent daily mind–body practice that if I didn't I would not be able to function as my best self. It's simply essential for my inner balance and resilience to keep a handle on my 'wound-up', perfectionist nature so it stays on the side of helpful and doesn't sabotage my bounce-back ability.

Moody Warriors

Moody warriors struggle with maintaining a positive, balanced mood. Everyone's mood balance fluctuates to some degree over time and life circumstances, but some people have what can be thought of as a lower mood 'set point' than others. If you have issues with low mood, depression and mood disorders running in your family, this tends to make you more likely to also have a challenge in this same area. However, even if this is the case for you, struggling with low mood is not a set-in-stone-for-life fixed point. Your mood set point can be shifted on a brain level over time using a variety of 'mood resilience tools' which we'll explore in Chapter Two. This ability to shift mood has been proven in brain-imaging studies on depression as well as many other types of research measuring mood over time.

Moodiness can show up in diverse ways. Some moody types can relate to looking at life through the 'glass half-empty' filter. Or you may be less consciously aware of your moods until they start to negatively affect your personal relationships, work or social life. For example, feeling irritable and on edge or, at the opposite end, withdrawn and un-social are all ways a moody warrior tends to cope with stress when they are out of balance, leading to more bad or low moods and fewer happy ones over time.

The reason balancing mood is so important for resilience is that when the brain and mind get stuck in the negative, our brain wiring can start to change too and get stuck. According to some imaging studies, the left front brain can start to become underactive or sluggish. Essentially, the brain goes into 'withdraw and protect' mode and can get really stuck in this 'brain avoidance' pattern. This is something that we see when we brain-map people suffering with depression or chronic low moods. This is the brain mode that dominates when we don't feel safe, and is meant to be protective. However, in modern life it causes a maladaptive low mood issue or, at its most severe, depression. This brain response may have served a more adaptive purpose – for example, in the caveman days when the brain activated this mode in the dead of winter to keep us indoors in the long, cold, dark nights, or after an injury so we stayed inside the cave and didn't venture too far afield before we recovered physically. Back then, most of the threats we faced were sudden, immediate, acute and physical dangers, not the chronic mental low-grade dangers of modern life that can trigger the same brain response, especially if you are genetically susceptible to low moods.

Often people may not meet the full criteria for depression, but feel like they have struggled in this positive mood area for many years or even most of their lives but just managed to 'get on with it'. However, it is completely possible to shift these patterns in the brain with specific easy practices such as simple loving-kindness meditations. These practices have been shown on brain-imaging studies to light up brain areas associated with positive moods and empathy. I often get asked if it is possible to shift out of low moods and moodiness even if you have an incurable or chronic health problem. The answer is yes, and this has again been proven in multiple research studies on resilience in people who have suffered from serious medical conditions including cancer and heart attacks. Those who are able to maintain their positivity despite these major traumatic health events have better health outcomes over time. For example, these positive patients lived longer, with a higher quality of life, even when the researchers controlled for other factors like smoking, bad diet or exercise.

Exhausted Warriors

This resilience type's main challenge is regulating their energy levels on a brain, cellular and body level. Everyone has their own unique energy set point, which is a combination of our genes and environment over time. Some of us may really need at least nine hours of sleep each night to feel optimally rested (I am one of those people!), while for others seven hours is still peachy as long as the sleep is good quality. If this is your resilience type, you are more likely to exceed your energy set point when you get out of balance, meaning your 'energy out' is bigger than your energy-making capacity.

Exhausted warriors are most likely to experience issues such as burnout, chronic fatigue, and feeling 'tired but wired', where you are drained but can't sleep. They may feel sluggish yet on edge during the day, and often wake up feeling unrested even after a full night's sleep.

Another indicator of an exhausted warrior is that you are always getting sick, taking longer to recover after a bug, have a lowered immunity to infections, immune dysfunction or autoimmune issues.

The immune system is very closely connected to our cell energy powerhouses, the mitochondria, and how well they are working can also affect our immune-system function. That is something we didn't know fifteen years ago in medicine when I was still in my doctor training years. Malfunctioning mitochondria seems to go along with malfunctioning immune-system function, according to a growing body of research.[1,2,3,4]

What this means is that things that affect our energy can impact our immune system too.

Once you know this is your resilience type, you can start giving your mitochondria and energy system a bit of extra support, understanding and nurturing. It also may not always be possible to get your optimal nine hours of sleep (hello, being a new parent or working shifts!) because in real life things are not always perfect. However, once you are aware of your needs, you can recognize the signs of fatigue sooner and manage your energy reserves to the best of your ability with the things you can control. For example, if you are not able to currently get your optimal sleep time each night, now is probably not the time to start training for a half-marathon or going on a strict weight-loss diet. In fact, putting yourself under more energy pressures when you are already not feeling your energetic best is one of the most common patterns I see in patients who come to see me with severe burnout and chronic fatigue spectrum illnesses. Often the trigger for their illness started after pushing themselves harder when they were already starting to feel tired and sluggish over a period. Frequently an autoimmune disease illness will first pop up after a period of mental and/or physical chronic overexertion or high stress which ends in exhaustion.

Many integrative practitioners who focus on mind–body medicine will also often say that they find their clients and patients who end up with these chronic low-energy and immunity issues are often 'helper personalities'. This is a personality trait that tends to put others before yourself, be a caregiver or nurturer, the friend or family member everyone else leans on. That can often lead to the energy-depletion issue over time because your own energy needs become secondary to everyone else's.

Scattered Warriors

The ability to focus, concentrate, think and make decisions clearly and having a solid memory are key factors for peak mental performance and are also keys to resilience. Scattered warriors are people who are out of balance in their ability to focus on the task at hand. They may feel overwhelmed and like they never quite catch up.

When our brains are stuck in distraction mode, or have trouble retaining new information (a brain skill called memory consolidation), it is very difficult to make traction in our daily life activities. The distraction makes it really hard to stick to even quite simple daily routines, habits and practices without getting derailed and feeling bad about it (leading to the procrastinate-then-feel-guilty cycle). These overlapping abilities to focus, have clarity of thought and retain new information are all needed to help you execute your life's vision. You need to have a clear head and focused mind to stay on track doing the little daily things that get you where you want to go in different aspects of your life, all while managing the daily stressors that can get in the way.

When I work with patients and clients who suffer with ADHD (or similar symptoms of feeling scattered, even without a medical diagnosis), they often have trouble remembering daily routines, tasks, personal commitments and following through with those commitments and obligations, despite their best intentions. Their memory for routine, boring things gets worse under stress too, to a greater extent than the other resilience types. This can put a huge strain on their relationships, which can impact things like social resilience (having a strong social-support network) and also mental and emotional health and resilience.

There is some very preliminary research to suggest that people with ADHD, the medical, more severe end of 'scattered', may also have trouble managing oxidative, or cell stress in the brain. This 'stress forgetfulness' often causes strain in both professional and personal relationships.

Related to this area of focus and clarity too are some very practical skills, like the ability to stay organized. This applies to organizing your thoughts as well as your environment – when these are 'tidy', they free up mental headspace too.

It is very common for scattered warriors to have lots of innovative ideas and a fast-paced mind, two things that can be a great asset for the creative process. On the flip side, this high-speed mind can contribute to the issue of starting many projects in the initial 'excitement' phase but becoming overwhelmed with the number of balls in the air. This leads to not being able to finish things once the brain gets a bit bored of them or when 'stress forgetfulness' starts to make following through more difficult.

Many if not most successful entrepreneurs are likely to be scattered types. Otherwise they never would have left their regular safe jobs and guaranteed salaries for the unknown. Scattered warriors take more risks, tend to be more adventurous and also need more reward and stimulation to keep them motivated. The danger, however, if this tendency is not managed well, is going down the road of constant distractibility, being unable to complete things on time, having trouble making decisions (i.e. procrastination and indecisiveness) and starting many things at once.

If this is your type, you also probably tend to be bold but also get bored easily, which can then show up in relationships and cause havoc in your personal life, especially if you were previously unaware of this tendency. When at your best, however, you can be massively creative and come up with novel solutions to problems.

This resilience type may also be more likely to have addictive tendencies, ranging from food addiction to substances or even shopping, to achieve that hit of brain reward chemicals, so this is something that is always worth keeping an eye on. Focusing that energy into positive activities such as Ironman endurance sports, jogging or ashtanga yoga can help funnel this obsessive tendency in a positive direction.

Scattered types also tend to prefer more 'extreme' strategies, whether it comes to diet, exercise or lifestyle changes. This can be a good thing if it helps you kickstart a health change, such as a healthier diet or exercise regimen, but it can also tip over into extremism that is nearly impossible to keep up, resulting in a 'stop–start' cycle and causing a lot of frustration. It can also lead to starting many wellness interventions or 'health kicks' at once and becoming overwhelmed by them so that you are not able to continue with any of them in the longer term.

Daily routines and rituals are especially important for scattered warriors, to give structure and predictability to the day and avoid confusion or distraction. This includes blocking out work, meals, wake-up, morning and bedtime routines around the same time each day and having a plan for getting back on track if things get off-schedule for a few days – say, on a weekend.

Scattered types have the tendency to get overwhelmed and even 'paralysed' by too many choices. This choice paralysis is compounded by the high degree of choice that modern life presents to us in nearly every aspect, from messaging apps, productivity tools, diets and supplements, to meditation, yoga and exercise classes. Breaking this choice paralysis is very important for enhancing resilience for scattered types. This paralysis causes a lot of stress and even anxiety, which both decrease resilience and can cause further imbalances.

The Resilience Spectrum

Finding your resilience type is just the first step in getting your bounce back. I have also discovered, while treating countless patients, that resilience is a spectrum. As well as helping my patients identify their resilience type, I also assess them with a resilience spectrum test.

We all move up and down the resilience spectrum depending on our circumstances, which means that at different times our needs change. What works for you today in terms of building your resilience may not work for you in a year's time when perhaps your job has changed or you are facing a health challenge.

The Resilience Spectrum Score

To calculate your Resilience Spectrum score, return to the Resilience Types quiz on page 16 and add up your total score (adding together the numbers for A, B, C and D). The maximum possible score is 180, but no one ever gets the perfect score so don't beat yourself up for being lower. And obviously the minimum score is 0, but I have never yet met that patient.

This score is a way of seeing where you are right now along the resilience spectrum. For example, you may be a moody warrior as your type, but in general you are only a teeny bit moody and mainly in balance, so your resilience score is high. Or, on the other hand, you might be a moody warrior who is really struggling and is in the 'code red' zone on the low end of the spectrum right now. It's all OK, because this score is just for you to get an idea of how things are going at the moment. In the pages that follow, you will get a resilience plan to help you start moving yourself up that resilience spectrum based on key practices, tips and habits for your type.

SCORE 140–180

Resilience Rock Star: You are rocking your resilience big time and are in the ultra-blue zone. Your protective factors are high, making you highly buffered against toxic stress effects. Your work is to look at the tips for your type in each area of the toolbox in Part Two and see where you want to focus your energies next to feel even more resilient. Being prepared for life's inevitable curveballs is about being ahead of the game.

SCORE 100–139

Steady Eddy: Your resilience is good, but there are likely to be some changes you can make to feel even better, based on your type and the imbalances you may be prone to under stress. The tools in Part Two will help you identify these and manage them.

SCORE 51–90

Code Yellow: Your resilience is on the low end, with several clear warning signs. So now's the time to make a move to avoid total stress, overwhelm or constantly feeling tired, anxious, down or foggy, depending on your type. It is the perfect opportunity to start some small changes in each area of the toolkit, like a five-minute mind–body practice, adding a power plant like CBD and/or making a food change like cutting out refined sugar for a while to start bringing you back into balance

SCORE: 0–50

Code Red: Your resilience is low, and you are at the highest level of vulnerability. You may be quite overwhelmed, but have faith: even one small lifestyle change can start moving you out of the red zone. When you are in 'code red' you may have multiple symptoms and it's hard to know where to start. Start with the tips for your main type and don't add to your overwhelm by trying to change too many things at once. Start with focusing on sleep for your main type in Part Two.

On the red end of the spectrum, when our resilience is lowest, we can become victims of toxic stress and feel powerless to change things. When in this red zone, we are most vulnerable to resilience zappers, like sources of physical or mental stress, and can feel really fatigued, even if you are not an exhausted warrior. For example, catching every single bug that's going, or struggling to find the energy for our everyday life. I have spent a lot of my medical career helping people in the red zone: those who suffer with chronic serious issues like PTSD, depression and anxiety, chronic fatigue syndrome, insomnia, women's health issues, autoimmune disease, people living with severe chronic pain and, most recently, Long Covid syndrome. All of these issues are huge challenges to our resilience. But even if you suffer with one (or many!) of these, it is still possible to shift out of the toxic-stress victim zone, enhance your resilience and shift your quality of life, energy levels and sense of wellbeing. Living with chronic medical conditions doesn't make you doomed to low resilience and constant suffering, even when a cure for your condition may not be possible with current medical therapies. Once you know your resilience type, you can use the resilience medicine principles to help find your hidden superpowers, as well as target your challenge areas. It is not always possible to permanently cure complex conditions such as chronic neurological pain or autoimmune disease, but it *is* completely achievable to lessen symptoms and suffering, to enhance quality of life and to regain a sense of control so that your illness doesn't run your life and sabotage your potential for happiness.

In the middle of the spectrum is what I call the 'I'm fine zone' where a lot of people I encounter also spend most of their time. This is the person who's at risk for things like burnout, feels a bit numb and just stuck 'on a treadmill' of existence, often just surviving their 9 to 5 or daily routine without a ton of joy or passion. In this zone, it's often hard to take action because nothing is really 'wrong' *per se* but life is not amazing either. The person in this category often comes to see me after they have had a fleeting 'Aha!' moment at a meditation class, retreat or after a 'magic-mushroom'/psilocybin or other form of psychedelic trip. They say they feel like they 'woke up' to the fact that they felt their current life was 'meh' most of the time and now wanted or even craved more out of life. The people who came to me for help with these things did so because they felt that part of their answer to breaking the 'just OK' feeling cycle was changing their health in some way. For some it was stopping weekend binge drinking or emotional eating. For others, it was learning how to cope with stress in a new way to replace the glass of wine and emotional-shutdown strategy that was making them feel stuck or numb. Resilience is more than the absence of disease or illness, it's also about creating a life you are excited and passionate about and freeing yourself from inner doubts or fears that may be holding you back from your best life.

On the blue 'ultra-resilient' end of the spectrum are those who feel they are living their best life, who can savour the present, find joy and fulfilment in their daily life, have access to their creativity and feel generally connected to their 'best selves'. They bounce back quickly from life's inevitable setbacks, stronger than before, without experiencing a major health breakdown. When people on this end of the resilience spectrum come to see me, they are often looking to expand creatively, or reach new heights of achievement in a specific area of their life. In some cases, they want to feel a greater internal sense of calm and contentment that may have eluded them despite massive personal and/or professional life success. Being in the blue zone of the resilience spectrum is also about being able to maintain your sense of inner balance and control, and return to it when things get off track. This is often known as having an 'internal locus of control' by scientists, meaning that *you* happen to your world rather than feeling that the world is happening *to* you as a passive observer. People who have mastered this internal locus of control or inner balance are far less likely to feel hopeless, despairing and helpless in the face of adversities and tend to bounce back much faster. In case you're wondering, let me reassure you that people in the blue zone don't have perfect health or medical histories. They can have chronic issues too, just like everyone else, but they have perfected the art of bouncing back and enhancing their quality of life despite their challenges.

Because we are complicated human beings who can't be easily divided into neat categories, you may find that in some elements of life you are in the blue resilience zone (crushing it with your career!) but in other areas (maybe health or relationships) you may be in the red or somewhere in the middle. That is the way it is with pretty much all of us and means you are both normal and human.

I often tell my patients when we work together on their resilience that the only entities that can stay constantly in the blue 'ultra resilience' or 'thrive' zone in *all* aspects of life *all* of the time are robots, not living, breathing human beings. Social media may want us to believe otherwise, but no one has a perfect day every day, and no one feels super-resilient all of the time. It's normal and natural for us to have times when we feel vulnerable, out of control, have self-doubt and even have blips of feeling helpless or hopeless. Try to embrace those moments and parts of yourself as much as the more resilient bits. I have discovered that, once you get into your resilience groove, these low bits don't last nearly as long or feel nearly as dire as they may have once felt, as your inner balance improves and makes it easier to get back on track.

Working with What You've Got

One of the themes I have found, working with many patients struggling with their resilience over the years, is that those who are struggling the most are often, paradoxically, doing the *most* work to try to get better. It is *so* frustrating! They tell me that the fact that they have had to devote every bit of mental and physical energy to their problems has made them even more depressed/anxious/exhausted/confused, since it seems like nothing seems to work despite their best efforts. This is where knowing your type comes in handy because if you are doubling down on what you may think is your perfect diet/meditation or other favourite wellness routines, thinking that you just have to do them all a bit harder, but still not getting results, you are probably doing the wrong things, or at least the less optimal things for your type.

I find these patients have no problem whatsoever listing all the things they have 'done wrong', the challenges they have and their failures. They very rarely, however, have thought much about what is right about themselves, what they are good at or looked with a curious eye at the strengths they already possess but may have overlooked or disregarded as 'not important'. When I ask about what they love, what they are great at, what makes them special or what brings them joy, they often look at me blankly, as life has often become 100 per cent about 'self-improvement', which isn't a particularly joyful way to live!

Growing our resilience is as much about finding our strengths and joys, working with rather than against ourselves, as it is about improving the weaker bits. When we are aware of our strengths and positive attributes, it is much easier to stay afloat mentally and emotionally – especially in a rough patch when we can focus on what is already right with us too. This way of approaching life, flowing with what is already good, gives our brain much-needed positive feedback which can create biological change in the brain and body.

So keep this in mind now that you have your score and your resilience type. You may have found out you are a focusing ninja (definitely not scattered!) but struggle with moodiness. Or that you are generally quite happy and social most of the time but tend to experience worry and anxiety quite regularly (i.e. the 'wound-up type').

The other thing to remember is that the quiz and the spectrum are simply a framework to assist you, so don't get caught up in the numbers too much. If your total resilience score is low right now, don't panic, because it's all shiftable. It is, however, useful to have *some* system to bring us awareness around our personal resilience. The human brain loves and seeks out systems, order and knowing 'where things are at'. That's just how we are wired because it helps us make sense of the world. Our brains also like tracking things and get a hit of feel-good chemicals when we can see objectively that something is improving over time. The world of resilience is huge, but my hope is that these tools are a helpful way to help you navigate your journey within it.

So just by discovering your type you have already taken the first step to becoming more resilient by understanding what makes you tick.

IMMUNE SYSTEM ISSUES AND CHRONIC
MEDICAL CONDITIONS

Many chronic health conditions involve a dysregulated nervous system and immune system and can cause overwhelm if you try to do too much too quickly. Conditions like this that I regularly treat in my medical practice include autoimmune diseases, chronic Lyme Disease and chronic fatigue syndrome or ME, chronic pain conditions, fibromyalgia and something called mast cell activation syndrome or MCAS, just to name a few. If you are working with one of these health issues or a similar one, being gentle with yourself and moving slowly is really important to building your resilience up slowly and surely, to avoid overwhelming or overly stressing the nervous system, which can result in setbacks. Start with your main type, but if you start to feel overwhelmed or exhausted you can also use the practices and recommendations for exhausted warriors too.

In addition to using this system, there are things like functional medicine testing and even some specific medications you may want to explore with your health practitioner that can help, based on my experience treating my own patients with these complex conditions successfully over many years.

The other piece of good news about resilience is that even if, like many of my patients, you suffer with complex chronic medical conditions that do not have a permanent cure, going on your resilience journey can help you take more control over your symptoms, bring in more joy, more energy and generally positive life experiences so you do not feel like you are defined solely by your illness or current limitations.

Overcoming Resilience Roadblocks

The most amazing part about resilience is your potential to get more of it regardless of what current challenges you face. In fact, the only true resilience roadblocks I have encountered are not any particular medical condition but are instead common thinking errors, or mental traps. I come across these regularly when I first start working with people on their resilience journey, no matter how intelligent or well-versed they are in health and wellness. My patients are often very aware of what healthy living looks like, and yet they aren't so clear about what healthy thinking is, and how unhealthy mental habits can undo so much of their good work. These are all totally normal reactions to change, so don't feel bad if you find yourself identifying with at least one or two of them.

I find that the most comment mental traps I see in my practice can be broken down as follows:

- **Over-intellectualizing**
  Over-analysing every detail to delay actually taking action. Thinking that simply talking about the theory of resilience will change you rather than committing to taking action. This is a super-tempting habit because committing to making changes in your lifestyle, food, habits, etc. creates discomfort at first, and even anxiety temporarily in the brain. It is easier to think about change than do it, and many people get stuck in the theory and don't actually make the changes they need. It can really feel like running uphill. This is totally normal, but don't worry, you can take things slow. Just make a few small changes at a time, using a minimal amount of time each day.

- **Thinking 'All I need is a holiday'**
  Everyone does need vacations and taking a holiday is definitely healthy and good for your overall resilience. However, just taking a vacation will not up your resilience factor in the long term. Normally people who rely on taking vacations to feel better

temporarily will feel less stressed on the trip and for a few days or a week after they return. But then the stress levels quite quickly get back up to pre-vacation levels because the underlying resilience roadblocks are not addressed. So it's a vicious 'living for the next vacation' cycle and it's super-common with my clients (who of course really struggled in the pandemic when that stress-buster was no longer available). The solution is growing your resilience in normal everyday life so you can enjoy those vacations for their own sake, rather than as a 'fix'. It's all about bringing back the daily joy in your 9 to 5, whether that is spent as a stay-at-home mum or working in the corporate world.

- **Thinking you must 'go it alone'**
  This is a common defence mechanism to help protect ourselves from rejection or the fear of embarrassment of sharing our struggles or challenges with our support network, which can be friends and family and also professionals like therapists, coaches or a doctor trained in these areas (e.g. an integrative medicine doctor, or integrative psychiatrist). Just like it takes a village to raise a child, as the saying goes, resilience also takes a village, meaning you need to create your own tribe of people to help support you on your resilience journey – family, friends, doctors, therapists, etc. You may be saying 'Wait, you just said I should be finding my own power and inner resilience, not waiting for someone to do it for me.' But building your team isn't relinquishing your power. In fact, it's empowering because you are choosing the people who are going to be best at supporting your resilience, while *you* are the one doing the work.

- **Convincing yourself the time isn't right**
  I hear so often from patients that they don't have time to address their resilience, or now is not the right time/I need to wait till the timing is better/I'll do it later. This is a very common rationalization for putting off making a change till some time in the future, and this rationalization can feel very convincing to your brain. It

can show up differently for different resilience types. For example, scattered warriors can tell themselves they are waiting for the perfect time and being able to get the perfect plan in place, and that before that happens it's not worth starting to make changes because they 'won't last'. For wound-up warriors, there is often anxiety about change. For moody warriors, getting and maintaining the motivation is the hardest part; and for exhausted warriors, it's too tiring. But fear not, by following the resilience programme for your type, you will be able to overcome these common roadblocks that everyone has in some shape or form when they start to work on their resilience.

- **Feeling 'Fake Good' or saying 'I'm Fine'**
  This is most common with wound-up warriors, who feel uncomfortable admitting they are not OK or asking for help, or feel guilty because they're not 'really' sick. They often just go, go, go till they totally burn out and end up in a stress crisis. You don't have to always be OK all of the time. It's normal and necessary to have an off day (or week!) and be honest about it. In fact, it's a key ingredient in building a more resilient you, taking the time you need to recover and rejuvenate, especially if you are an exhausted warrior.

So now you know your resilience type and where you are right now on the resilience spectrum and how to spot any resilience roadblocks to move them out of your path. Next, we will learn about the science and biology of resilience and what makes you tick when it comes to resilience in the brain and body.

CHAPTER TWO

THE SCIENCE OF RESILIENCE

When I was a junior doctor, one of my favourite treatments to administer was removing ear wax or, as it's called officially, 'impacted cerumen removal'. This wasn't because it was particularly challenging or glamorous, it was quite the opposite. You basically take a huge metal water-filled plunger, warm up the water to a nice temperature and, after looking inside the blocked ear canal, gently squirt water in there to dislodge the wax. We even used to provide patients with a barber's cape to prevent their clothing from getting wet because the water usually got everywhere. It wasn't a high-tech procedure by any means, it was quite a humble, basic thing. But the reason why it was my favourite when I first started out as a doctor was because it was one of the only situations in family medicine where a patient could walk in with a major issue (not being able to hear properly) and walk out happily 'cured', even if temporarily. It made people so happy. I felt like when I had a patient booked for this, I could guarantee I would make at least one person's day happier in under five minutes.

This procedure, with its immediate and happy outcome, became a highlight of my junior-doctor workdays because most of the time my patients were suffering from chronic, complex conditions where there was no quick fix or cure in the western-medicine drugs toolkit. I learned that the only way to get relief from many, if not most, of these chronic symptoms was by using a multi-pronged integrative approach that, over time, impacts resilience on a brain, mind and body level.

The results of this kind of integrative practice may not be immediate, but I can promise you that building true and lasting resilience is powerful medicine, and it's a medicine that everyone can access, tune into and benefit from, no matter what their circumstances. When we develop resilience, we don't do it just to get rid of a particular health symptom, but to master stress and live a happier life. Thanks to modern science, we now are able to begin to untangle and understand many of the resilience factors inside of each of us and how we can activate our 'adaptive magic'.

Resilience Starts in the Brain

We exist in a state of dynamic equilibrium, or shifting balance, between stresses to our system and resilience factors to help buffer them. The brain is the master control switch for overall resilience, impacting everything from our immune function, mood balance and digestion to our body's hormone balance, including our stress hormone cortisol, as well as our 'softer' resilience skills like mental and emotional balance. In medicine, doctors tend to separate the brain from the body because that's how the medical system works: neurologists will focus on 'brain factors' in isolation, while hormone specialists (endocrinologists) will focus on 'body hormones' despite these two systems interacting to a huge degree, both influencing the balance between 'bad stress' or resilience.

In reality, the brain and body are in continuous, constant communication through our chemical-messenger systems, hormones, immune cells in our blood and body fluids and our nerve cells. The way the brain perceives stress is one of the main determinants of our overall resilience. The brain, not the adrenal glands where stress hormones get made, is actually the key organ of the stress response. This may be surprising to many. However, the reason why the brain is the trump card is because it is the brain, not the adrenal gland or any other organ, that determines what is stressful or represents a 'threat' and then orchestrates the brain and body response accordingly. The cool part is that in order to build resilience, we actually need stress, since resilience is the adaptive-magic part that happens as a result of experiencing stress. So again, no need to worry about trying to avoid or 'get rid of' stress triggers entirely. It's more about turning the stress from feeling toxic to our brain to something of a positive challenge, as we will see.

When I ask a new patient 'What do you feel is the biggest barrier for you right now?' a few common themes pop up:

- 'My memory is not as good as it used to be' – Scattered
- 'I feel so tired after work that I don't have the energy for the things I would like to do' – Exhausted
- 'I always feel switched on, I can't relax even on the weekend' – Wound-up
- 'I can't fall asleep easily at night or stay asleep, even if I am really tired' – Wound-up
- 'I have a mystery health problem with loads of weird symptoms that the doctors can't seem to fit together' – Exhausted
- 'I just can't seem to focus and the harder I try to force it, the more it escapes me and I feel totally frustrated' – Scattered
- 'I'm just in survival mode' – all types, but most often Exhausted and Moody
- 'I feel like I've lost my mojo, there's no joy in my life' – Moody

These issues share a common theme. They are all markers of dysregulated brain–body communication and an imbalance between resilience promoters and resilience zappers. This imbalance starts at a brain level with not being able to shut off the stress response when it is no longer adaptive or necessary. So again, it's an issue with the response to stress, not the stress event itself that needs solving.

We now know from recent research that stress in the brain affects each of us a bit uniquely, depending on things like your resilience type and other factors like our genes and environment. Brain stress gone wrong may derail your digestion or affect your mood or even your hormone levels. Often a combination of things go wrong in the brain, leading to many confusing symptoms that don't seem to fit under one single illness or diagnosis. It's just a giant ball of stress-related symptoms that are very real, but without one easy fix.

Because the brain and body (including the gut, which acts as a 'little brain') are so connected, brain and nervous-system overwhelm and dysregulation lead to problems that can show up anywhere in the body. Many patients experiencing these issues are told by their doctors that they have a 'mystery illness'. But when you see the symptoms through the lens of brain stress running amok without appropriate resilience mechanisms, that mystery diagnosis doesn't seem so mysterious after all.

If this sounds familiar, don't worry. Even if brain stress has been wreaking havoc on your resilience for months or even years, it's never too late to break the cycle feeding these issues and get more resilient by working with your type. But before we get into how to fix things in Part Two, we will learn a bit more about the biology of resilience and how it all relates to your type.

It's Not Just 'All in Your Head'

For years I have focused my medical practice on people suffering with what has previously been called 'psychosomatic' symptoms: ranging from all-over body pain that tends to move around the body, to brain fog, overwhelm, anxiety and many other stress-related symptoms as well as gut disorders such as irritable bowel syndrome. Until recently, these disorders were believed by most doctors to be 'mental' disorders and patients suffering with them were often, unfairly, deemed 'problem patients' or 'untreatable', or blamed for having 'difficult personalities'.

However, I have found that far from being untreatable or being 'personality issues', these are very real symptoms with a biological basis, even if we don't understand every exact mechanism yet. These symptoms can be successfully treated and improved with an integrative medicine approach focused on enhancing resilience from all angles and tailoring the plan to the person's resilience type among other factors.

These symptom clusters are now understood to have a biological basis related to a combination of factors including inflammation inside our cells, gut-microbiome issues called 'dysbiosis' and increased oxidative-stress (cell-stress) vulnerability as well as multiple brain changes due to chronic unchecked stress on top of a genetic predisposition.

Due to the two-way crosstalk between the brain and body, psychological interventions such as meditation, as well as biological therapies such as a resilience diet, supplements, gut-microbiome healing protocols, medical cannabis and certain medications that work on the immune system, all play a role in helping us heal from these disorders. While there is no single overnight quick fix, all of these interventions enhance our resilience in different ways, creating a snowball effect of becoming more and more resilient over time, decreasing chronic symptoms and improving holistic health. These simple interventions work best when tailored to your type and your lifestyle too.

If you have scored on the high end of the resilience spectrum, have perfect health and are reading this book to take your resilience to the next level, these principles may feel less urgent. But applying them can prevent an issue from starting in the first place, as well as helping you to feel even better and supercharge your strengths.

Our Stress Response and Resilience

The way we respond and react on a brain level to stress is central to determining how resilient we are. And sometimes our brain does the 'wrong' thing in the context of what is necessary for modern life. We evolved to be able to mount a stress response to save us as cavemen from sudden or 'acute' dangers, such as helping our ancestors get the rush and spurt of energy they needed to run away from a predator. In modern life, there are fewer acute threats in daily life but almost countless sneaky 'chronic' or daily small mental threats. But our fight-or-flight response system still operates like it did when we were living in caves. Our brains still respond to these daily mental threats as they would to a threat to our physical safety – it sees them as 'mental predators' lying in wait. Our fight-or-flight system is actually very complex, but one of the simplest models and important parts of it is something called the HPA Axis – which stands for the hypothalamic–pituitary–adrenal axis. This is the system involving parts of the brain that talk to our adrenal glands (that make our stress hormones) and it controls our stress or fight-or-flight response. This is not the whole picture, but it is a good model to explain why and how bad stress can really mess with your resilience when it gets out of hand.

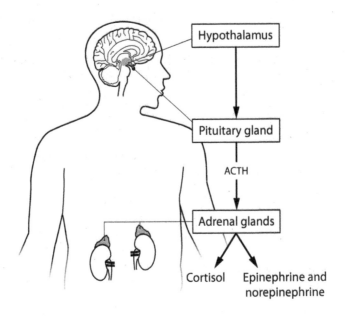

What happens when *any* threat is detected is our brain's hypothalamus sends a signal to the adrenal glands (which sit on top of our kidneys) to make more cortisol, our stress hormone. In an ideal world this stress response should die down after the threat passes, like it used to when the predator was gone and we went back to our cave relaxed and relieved: no more cortisol stress hormone getting pumped out! However, the small mental threats we experience are, unlike a predator, constant and unrelenting in modern life. So we keep making more stress hormone every time a small thing triggers the system, from that stressful email to constant social-media notifications, messaging-app alerts and other distracting things competing for our attention. It's not just cortisol that's released, but many other brain chemicals and inflammatory mediators, creating a 'stress soup' in the brain and body.

The problem with this for our modern lives is that the stress and cortisol response is only adaptive (i.e. healthy and helpful) when it comes on briefly to help us fight a physical threat and then goes away. If the stress hormone levels stay high and become chronic (i.e. they remain high all the time or for days on end), this starts to damage us, our brains and even our immune system and gut health. Our biology hasn't yet adapted fully to the small but constant mental threats of modern life. Chronic brain exposure to higher cortisol levels also lowers neuroplasticity,[1] or your brain's ability to change itself and adapt.

The fight-or-flight system, or sympathetic nervous system (SNS) is a part of the nervous system known as the autonomic nervous system (ANS). The ANS is exactly like it sounds – it operates automatically to help balance stress and regulate normal non-stress body and brain functions like resting, digesting and thinking clearly. We don't have to think about these bodily functions, they just happen for us.

The ANS has two arms that have to be in balance for optimal resilience: the SNS, which handles the stress and danger alarm system, ramping up our response to threats, and the parasympathetic nervous system, or PNS. The PNS is the arm of the nervous system involved in calming things down so that we don't get stuck in that hyperarousal, jacked-on-stress, high-cortisol state long term.

It is easy to think *OK, that must mean SNS bad, PNS good*, but that is an oversimplification. We need *both* arms of the nervous system in order to function, and they are more like partners than opposites or enemies. It's the optimal balance of the two that is the key to resilience. We need both of them to function properly for everything from sleeping, breathing and keeping our hearts beating, to operating well under mental and physical pressures. This balance is dynamic and constantly changing or 'recalibrating' on a moment-to-moment basis. As is the theme with most resilience factors in the brain, flexibility in this balancing act is key – being able to tone down the fight-or-flight response to rejuvenate 'on demand'. A lack of this balance is linked to burnout and toxic stress overwhelm in multiple studies.

One of the main players in the PNS is a special nerve called the vagus nerve, which runs from the brain to the thorax, via your breathing muscle, the diaphragm. The vagus nerve helps counterbalance the stress response in the body by triggering a relaxation effect when it's activated. We can help to activate the vagus nerve through simple breathing exercises, which are explained in Part Two. The ANS and its two arms use brain neurochemicals and hormones to help regulate this balance, in a complex symphony of brain resilience.

When the ANS balance gets out of whack, problems start. Conditions as diverse as POTS (Postural Orthostatic Tachycardia Syndrome), where people get debilitating symptoms of dizziness, easy fainting and fatigue, and ADHD (which tends to affect scattered types most often) have been linked to ANS imbalances and instability, especially when faced with a stressor of any sort. Again, the good news is that these issues are in fact changeable over time and we can learn to balance our ANS as adults even if we didn't learn to do this in infancy and childhood (due to a combination of genes plus environment).

So we know that the way in which stress affects our resilience and nervous system can be shifted. What's even cooler is that our perception of how much stress is 'good' stress can also change too. Over a hundred years ago, two psychologists, Robert **Yerkes** and John **Dodson**, figured out that stress isn't necessarily bad for you. In fact, their research showed that some stress actually enhances our performance (by 'performance' they meant how well we can function mentally, emotionally and physically). It was discovered that some people could turn stress from a negative into a positive. Instead of stress chronically depleting them and leading to eventual exhaustion, the opposite happened: they seemed to bounce back better than before when something stressful happened. Their stress tolerance went up (aka, their resilience).

So what was their secret? What's the key to making stress positive and a resilience enhancer rather than a resilience killer? It's all about the amount of stress you feel on a brain level. How much stress we feel in the brain is subjective, meaning it's different for each of us. One person's overwhelmingly demanding day is another person's perfectly balanced day. Luckily stress is also something we can get some control over, using a variety of strategies you can tailor to your type. However, at the core of it, no matter what your type is, the skill of reframing stress is to see it as a challenge rather than a threat.

This mindset shift from threat to challenge changes how your brain and body perceive the stress and ultimately get less freaked out by it, meaning that the HPA axis and other brain stress areas don't go into overdrive chronically. One example would be finding out that you have pre-diabetes. This is news I often have to give to patients because it's something I screen for at my clinic. The first reaction from patients is naturally fear, maybe some disbelief and then feeling quite down about the fact that they have been told they are 'on their way' to having diabetes. Some patients visibly panic. However, another way of looking at this diagnosis would be as a positive challenge and opportunity to feel better: you have an opportunity to improve your blood-sugar control now, before things get worse, and the best news is that pre-diabetes is reversible with food and lifestyle change. Now that you know about your condition, you can prevent it from going any further. Even better, because of the healthy changes you will make, you will be the healthiest you've been in years and have much more energy and fewer food cravings than before.

Another example would be a mental stressor. Imagine that you have just found out that you are going to be made redundant in your job. Initially, you would worry about losing the comfortable job and income you have been used to. However, if you reframe this change as a positive challenge, maybe this is your opportunity to do something you are more passionate about, turn a part-time hobby into a more full-time gig, something you have been talking about doing for years but haven't quite managed to 'take the leap'.

Especially if you are a moody warrior, you may find this 'reframing' technique quite difficult at first. But the good news is that it gets easier the more you practise.

Another element in turning threats into positive challenges we can handle is physical factors. For example, if your body is depleted of a certain nutrient or needs some help in a particular area, adding a supplement that may help support cellular energy or the body's detoxification system may make you physically more resilient to stress too. How much 'help' we need in this physical or biological department is partly dependent on our genes as well as our life experiences that influence the genes we're born with.

Over time you can increase the amounts and types of stress your brain sees as a challenge (i.e. 'good stress') before it turns into perceiving them as a toxic threat (i.e. 'bad stress'). This is basically like helping your brain adapt its reactions to stress to modern life a bit better. This rule about stress was named after the researchers who discovered it and is called the Yerkes/Dodson Law.

RESILIENT APPROACH: Shift, expand your curve. Perform better under greater stress.

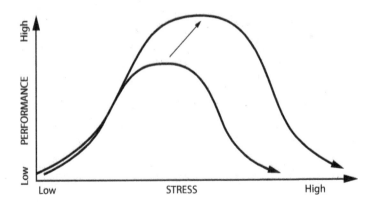

Source: *Yerkes Dodson.*

This model shows there is a level of stress which is required in which a person performs the best both mentally and physically. This sweet spot where stress is a good thing is what I like to call the 'thrive zone'. It's the spot where we still feel in control of the stress. The more resilient we become, the peak amount of stress that can still be 'good' stress increases, meaning we can handle more stress without it turning bad, becoming toxic or damaging us mentally or physically.

Starting to reframe our setbacks, bad news and adversity in terms of a challenge rather than a toxic threat is a skill that can be learned. It's not always easy, especially if you have had a string of bad luck or stressful things happening to you all at once, so it's important to be kind and patient as you do this. However, it is doable no matter how stressful things are right now. All mind–body practices help do this by helping tune up that SNS to PNS balance, and by choosing a practice that best suits your type, you can shift things most easily. You will be able to discover the best-fit practices for you in Part Two, in the mind–body chapter (page 181).

Threat Response (lowers resilience):	Challenge Response (boosts resilience):
Too much SNS activity	Optimal SNS:PNS balance
Blood vessels get smaller, blood flow and oxygen to the brain goes down (harder to think clearly, mental 'shutdown')	Blood vessels get wider, more oxygen and blood flow to brain to make the brain work better under pressure
Heart rate and blood pressure goes up – physically making us feel more stressed and panicky	Small burst of stress hormone, but then it drops back to normal – making us feel energized to take action and then returning us to a calm baseline
Stress hormone stays high – making us feel 'tired but wired' – and can lead to serious fatigue, especially for exhausted types	Positive emotions and mental patterns kick in, to focus the brain for action and 'reframe' setbacks into challenges that can be met successfully
Negative emotions and mental patterns kick in – gets you stuck in negative brain loops that make the threat seem even bigger especially if you are a moody type	Enhanced creative problem-solving ability and accurate thinking
Feel overwhelmed, pressurized	Feel energized yet focused
Loss of high-level decision-making and lateral thinking	
Decreased ability to focus	
Tendency to make knee-jerk decisions that may not be well thought out (especially if you are a scattered type)	

Threat v. Challenge Response and Resilience. This table shows what actually happens in the physical body and in the brain when something is detected as a 'threat' (which lowers our resilience) rather than as a 'challenge' (which increases resilience).

As you can see from this table, when the brain perceives something as a challenge, it sees an opportunity for growth or gain and kicks in with positive emotions as well as physical body markers of a healthy response to stress. The challenge is seen as 'good stress'. This happens when we feel like 'we got this' and the mind flips into focusing on the positive.

When the mind sees something as a toxic threat, often due to a lack of resilience resources, the brain and body go into 'protect and shut down' mode, with more negative emotions. The brain homes in on potential threats and focuses our attention on the negative. Those negative emotions can spiral fast into sadness, anger, hopelessness and a feeling of helplessness, especially if your resilience type is moody warrior.

Depending on your resilience type, there are specific simple mind–body techniques that can best help reframe the way your brain perceives threats and can help you reduce mental overwhelm. For example, if you are a wound-up warrior, learning how to avoid getting stuck in the wound-up 'stress-hyperarousal' state or 'brain-panic mode' as your default reaction to stress can help you reduce the sense of feeling on edge and always slightly overwhelmed.

The way we eat and supporting our stress response with cannabinoids and other natural supplements can also play a role, as we will learn in Part Two.

Improving your Relaxation Response

Helping your brain to change perceived threats into challenges and lower your total stress load need not take hours a day, nor does it have to be complicated. One of the simplest ways to reframe your response to stress is by starting to regularly access a natural brain and body state called the Relaxation Response or RR.

This RR is actually our inbuilt counterpart to the fight-or-flight system or sympathetic nervous system overdrive that causes a build-up of bad stress. The RR helps engage our parasympathetic nervous system and restore that autonomic nervous system balance we just learned about. This helps bring about true relaxation in the nervous system, which is not something that happens when most people think they are 'relaxing' by watching a movie or even going to a physical yoga class. Neither of these is truly relaxing if the mind is still running around while you watch a film or sweat through your poses.

The RR was discovered in the 1970s by renowned Harvard professor and doctor, author and researcher Dr Herbert Benson, who was also the founder of the world-leading Benson–Henry Institute for Mind Body Medicine Massachusetts General Hospital. I had the honour of studying mind–body medicine for physicians with Dr Benson a decade ago and learned firsthand from his over half a century of wisdom in this field.

This RR is actually an inbuilt resilience mechanism we are born with. But because of the frantic pace of modern life, the constant mental stimulation and distraction and the lack of instruction in these practices in places like school or at the doctor's surgery, most people are totally unaware of this mechanism we all possess to harness bad stress.

Dr Benson studied the RR for over forty years and noticed that people who were able to turn on their RR were less susceptible to the 'bad' type of stress – meaning that any stress didn't seem to affect them as much or 'stress them out'. In effect, the activated RR created a toxic-stress buffer zone for them.

It turns out that many mind–body practices can switch on our RR. Some of the ways of turning on our RR range from visualization techniques, to a variety of meditation techniques, tai chi and many forms of yoga, going for an acupuncture or therapeutic massage session, prayer and many breathing techniques. What these practices all have in common is that they decrease sympathetic nervous system arousal levels, lower our heart rate and blood pressure, and lead to a focused, calm mental state, free from worried mental background chatter. Part of making these practices a part of your life is finding the best technique or set of techniques you can do for even just a few minutes a day, based on your resilience type. You can find out which ones may suit you best in Part Two, in the mind–body chapter (page 181).

Generally, the wound-up warriors find activating their RR more challenging than other resilience types, but any type can find it tricky in the beginning because this is simply not a skill we learn in modern life normally. Matching the person to the practice helps remove barriers to not being able to access the RR easily.

Brain Wiring for Resilience

To recap, good stress is the sort that leads to the brain and body feeling challenged but not overwhelmed, interpreting stress as challenges that can be won successfully and mastered. Bad stress, on the other hand, leads to that horrible feeling of being constantly under pressure or 'stressed out'. This happens when experiences or stressors feel out of our control or ability to master, are prolonged, draining and exhausting.

So the main thing that determines whether stress is 'good' (i.e. leads to more resilience) or 'bad' (i.e. leads to depleting your resilience) is how your brain interprets it, which luckily we can shift over time using the resilience toolkit in Part Two.

Mind–body practices and small shifts in our beliefs and behaviour can have a direct impact on our brain's chemical balance (neurotransmitters), brain networks and even brain structure over time, to create more resilient brains. Our brains are flexible, or neuroplastic, so the good news is that we can train the brain to shift its perception of stress over time at any age.

Brain Resilience Areas

Just like there are 'stress circuits' that can decrease our resilience, there are also resilience circuits and areas of the brain too. Specific brain areas and brain patterns appear to be particularly important for resilience and countering those stress circuits in the limbic system. Most of these areas and patterns are involved with processing emotions as well as stress, but at a less 'knee-jerk' and more conscious level than in the limbic system. Two of these are brain regions called the PFC (prefrontal cortex) and more specifically within it, a sub-area called the vm (ventral medial) PFC.[2] When these areas are not activating properly or become inflexible, the brain has a harder time adapting and hence is more vulnerable to low resilience states (being on the red end of the resilience spectrum from earlier). However, when the PFC is working well, it helps integrate and sort through all the information coming into the brain and coordinate a calm, clear-headed response – keeping you 'cool as a cucumber' under pressure. Another resilience area called the dorsal anterior cingulate cortex (dACC) 'talks' to our amygdala to help buffer negative moods and depression.

So how does this help us practically? It turns out that these brain are as light up with many forms of meditation and mind–body practices, like the ones you'll learn to do in Part Two.

Another good piece of news, especially if you are a moody warrior, is that emotional and mood regulation tends to get better, according to some researchers, as we age. Meaning even if you have suffered for many years with your mood resilience, you are more likely to get better as you get older, especially if you are taking small steps to activate these networks over time.

Flexible Brains Are Resilient Brains

Brain imaging and EEG (electroencephalogram) brain-activity pattern studies, along with other brain imaging used in research, allow us to get a snapshot of some aspects of brain functioning. They confirm that one of the most important things for brain resilience is flexibility. This means the brain's ability to change itself and adapt to our environment under pressures and stresses. This ability to adapt and change over time and create new brain cells and brain networks is called neuroplasticity. Everyone's brain has this capability for flexible change. You can enhance it over time if yours is not particularly adaptive at the moment, using the tools for your type in Part Two. You are not stuck with the brain wiring you have today for ever.

There are a few typical brain-pattern issues that tend to plague each resilience type. For wound-up warriors, it's the inability to shut off constant mental worry and wind down. For mood warriors, it's being unable to break out of low moods. For exhausted warriors, it's the struggle to maintain energy levels; and for scattered warriors, it's being unable to achieve focused mental clarity. In each case, the brain can essentially become 'stuck' in certain functional and brain-wave patterns. When this happens, and certain patterns become wired in over time, the brain has a much harder time responding optimally to stress and learning new ways of coping as easily: it becomes more resistant to changing. This creates a vicious cycle as people then become less open to new ideas or ways of trying to break the cycle. So no matter what your kryptonite is, the key is knowing what sort of rut you may be most prone to so that you can take quite specific type-focused steps to bust out of it. In Part Two, you will learn to do just that, using the resilience toolkit.

This is also where therapeutic psychedelics can be very useful for helping 'unstick' unhelpful brain patterns, such as in treatment-resistant depression. The active ingredient in magic mushrooms, psilocybin, has been granted 'breakthrough' therapy status by the US FDA to help speed up its approval it for use with patients. It is being used in research studies here in the UK too, where it will very likely soon be legal as a medicine prescribed by a doctor. Ketamine, a very old drug used originally to put people to sleep for surgeries, is already being used for a similar purpose in conditions such as depression and chronic pain, to help 'shake up' dysfunctional brain patterns even when other methods have failed. These compounds are now being rebranded as 'fast-acting antidepressants' and one of the ways they work is by inducing neuroplasticity, helping break those ruts to stimulate novel thinking again and kick-start the brain's potential for resilience. It's one of the most exciting new frontiers of mental health.

The Emerging Science of Psychoneuroimmunology

In the past decade, there have been enormous medical advances in areas of neuroscience (brain science) and the immune system (immunology). One of the most profound discoveries has been that our immune systems, our brain-chemical systems (neurotransmitters) and our gut microbiome (our gut bacteria) are all connected. These are collectively sometimes known as 'the big three'.

Each of these three systems affects the others in ways that western medicine didn't think possible fifteen years ago. This ongoing dance between our brain, gut and immune system has a huge impact on our overall resilience. We cannot separate the mind from the body as we once thought we could. The factors which influence our mood are not just in the brain, nor is what influences our immune system only in our body. It's basically a brain–body–immune-system superhighway going on inside us.

Psychoneuroimmunology or PNI is defined as the evidence-based neuroscience, or brain science, behind the complex interactions among our emotions, behaviour, nervous systems, hormones and immune system. It explains a lot about how bad stress can impact our immune system, and it explains some of the very common issues I had noticed for years in my patients with chronic diseases. Patients who came to see me for chronic pain often also suffered from depression. Many also suffered terribly with fatigue. The same pattern of pain + fatigue + low mood is also very common in patients with autoimmune disorders like lupus, ankylosing spondylitis and rheumatoid arthritis. In short, chronic pain, autoimmune diseases and depression seemed to go together a lot of the time. It wasn't just that people felt down or depressed about the fact that they had a chronic disease, although that would certainly be understandable. I became convinced after speaking with thousands of my patients who suffered with these overlapping problems that there was also a biological reason too.

We now know that people who suffer with chronic pain, as well as autoimmune disorders, have increased levels of pro-inflammatory chemicals in their brain and body. People suffering with at least some types of depression as well as chronic fatigue syndrome also have increased levels of these same immune chemicals. Many drugs to treat both autoimmune diseases and depression work by decreasing these inflammatory cytokines. My favourite treatment for patients with a combination of pain, fatigue and depression, especially when other things have failed, is medical cannabis, which we believe works in part thanks to its anti-inflammatory effect. It may reduce the levels of these cytokines as well as impacting the endocannabinoid system, another balancing system that connects the brain, gut and immune system.

Understanding the link between the 'big three' is often a huge relief and 'Aha!' moment for many of my patients, who had been told their depression, fatigue or brain fog had 'nothing to do with' their autoimmune disease or their pain condition. This contradicted my patients' personal experience of noticing that when their pain or inflammation flared up, mood and energy crashes followed. This experience was often dismissed by their doctors, making them feel even more confused about their symptoms and their ability to know their body and take any control over things. When I explained the link, and that certain treatments ranging from cannabis to meditation and specific pre and probiotics could help their symptoms, in part at least by addressing inflammation and this immune-system–brain–body link, these patients had hope again. If you suffer from one or more of these issues, you will be able to use the resilience toolkit in Part Two to help address some of these inflammation drivers too.

Inflammation is not always a bad thing. In fact, in acute situations, it is a normal, adaptive immune-system stress response to try and promote healing after an accident or injury. For example, when you break your arm, an inflammatory response helps bring blood and immune cells to the area to start the bone-healing process.

However, where inflammation becomes a problem and turns bad is when it becomes chronic, or sticks around, or has an exaggerated response and the immune system goes overboard with the inflammation. Reducing this chronic or 'bad' inflammation is a major keystone to enhancing our overall resilience, based on the research evidence we have so far, as well as what I have seen in real life for thousands of patients and clients with these chronic conditions over the past ten-plus years of medical practice. We can do this, luckily, via an 'anti-inflammatory' programme, or a resilience programme, that looks again at foods, supplements, mind–body and physical-movement practices as the core pillars. You will learn about this in Part Two, and tailor it based on your type.

MICROGLIA – THE BRAIN IMMUNE CELLS AND BRAIN INFLAMMATION

Microglia are special immune cells in our brain and nervous system. They are involved with brain flexibility (neuroplasticity), making new brain cells (neurogenesis), regulating memory, mood and stress balance. Not much was known about them until quite recently, however we know now that they play a huge role in regulating the brain–immune-system axis and in neuro, or brain, inflammation. Normally when things are running smoothly in the brain and stress is under control, microglia are just chilling out in a nice calm, quiet state or, as scientists call it, 'quiescence'. However, their balance can be thrown off by a threat such as an infection, acute stress or other insult. This throws them into 'alarm' mode and they start releasing those inflammatory cytokine chemicals (such as IL-1β, TNF-α, IL-6, NO, PGE2 and superoxide). These are brain chemicals secreted by different brain cells and the immune system, including microglia, which then affect brain 'stress circuits'. This can start a cycle of damaging neighbouring brain cells, which then release more cytokines and produce more cell damage over time, increasing inflammation.

These microglia likely play a significant role in conditions such as chronic fatigue syndrome/ME, depression, fibromyalgia and Long Covid. Conventional antidepressants, old therapies (rarely used now) such as electric-shock therapy (ECT), a medication called LDN (low dose naltrexone) and psychedelics like the magic-mushroom extract all seem to work on these microglia in a positive way.[3] Other things like a ketogenic diet can make microglia function better (see Part Two of this book under resilience diet for details). Cannabinoids from the cannabis plant such as those found in medical cannabis and CBD wellness products also impact our microglia[4] and help calm them back down again. (See the endocannabinoid system section, page 56).

PNI and Stress

The growing body of evidence around psychoneuroimmunology also demonstrates that any form of stress, physical as well as psychological or mental, can have a massive effect on our immune system. Over time, chronic unchecked stress can sabotage immune function, leading to physical health problems and illness in the body.

Even more intriguing has been the recent discovery of special proteins inside our cells called 'inflammasomes' that can turn on the 'bad' kind of inflammation. Researchers are discovering that these inflammasomes are regulated by our immune system and can be turned on by mental stress in animal models. The theory is that mental stress is actually sensed by the innate arm of the immune system (the first line of immune defence) in the brain, turning on inflammasomes and triggering inflammation reactions.

There is lots of talk about an 'anti-inflammatory diet' being able to solve all of these inflammation issues on its own. Diet is indeed very important for resilience and different types may need slightly different things, as you will see in Chapter Four on food, but I have many patients who eat the so-called 'perfect' and 'clean' diet and still end up with autoimmune issues. The reason is that inflammation is a very complex reaction, so having that 'anti-inflammatory lifestyle' is really more accurate in terms of what makes the most impact, using a variety of tools for your type (see Part Two).

Part of this new field of psychoneuroimmunology is also the brain–gut connection. Stress plays a role in both leaky brain and leaky gut (see page 58 for more detail), which is where the intestinal barrier is impaired and becomes more permeable, meaning that material from the gut leaks into the bloodstream. This leakiness, we think, can lead to immune responses and inflammation in places they shouldn't be, contributing to a whole range of symptoms and issues in both the brain and body, ranging from chronic fatigue and brain fog to depression. So, as you can see, everything is indeed connected.

There was a time when we thought depression might be a straightforward 'serotonin-deficiency' issue, serotonin being one of the key brain chemicals that regulates mood. That theory is now outdated and overly simplistic. The reality is much more complex. Depression is an example of how inflammation and brain–immune-system cross talk impacts mental health and resilience – while moody warriors are most likely to experience depression, it can hit any resilience type.

Depression is used so often as a model for brain resilience because it is such a well-researched model of resilience v. vulnerability. Depression is also sadly incredibly common, especially if you include milder forms like chronically low moods. The full story of depression involves a complex cascade of multiple brain chemicals, inflammatory chemicals and at least in some types, inappropriate brain inflammation. So in fact depression, as well as virtually all mental-health diagnoses, likely involves the immune system too.

Not all 'depression' is caused by the same exact combination of brain factors, which is why the same medication and approach doesn't work for everyone. However, new 'fast-acting antidepressants' including psilocybin from magic mushrooms offer hope to those with 'treatment-resistant' depression as part of an integrative approach. They have a brain-protective effect and normalize the microglia faster and seem to work when conventional drugs don't, such as in treatment-resistant depression.[5]

I have also seen patients who had self-treated Long Covid symptoms, which now affects millions of people, successfully using microdosing with psilocybin. In our clinic, we are also now combining medical cannabis with other anti-inflammatory integrative medicine therapies, supplements and mind–body approaches to treat Long Covid using the PNI framework.

The bottom line here is that when we start to calm stressors and inflammation in the brain and body, our immune systems become happier and more resilient. This also works the other way: when we nourish ourselves with healthy foods, decrease environmental toxin exposures, support a healthy gut microbiome (good gut bugs) and utilize natural supplements effectively for our type when needed, our immune system works better to help us cope with the mental and physical stresses that life throws at us, leading to lower overall stress and inflammation and happier brains.

The Endocannabinoid System: The Master Resilience System

We also have a very special system in our brain and body called the ECS, or endocannabinoid system. This is our main balancing system that we use to maintain homeostasis or 'brain + body balance'. It helps to regulate everything from sleep–wake cycles to our stress response and inflammation control. I learned about this system in detail first hand from my patients over a decade ago, even before there was a ton of research. And it was all because of medicinal cannabis, since plant compounds such as CBD and THC work on this system we all have naturally too. CBD is the most common non 'psychotropic' plant chemical in the cannabis plant, meaning it won't make you feel high. THC is known as the chemical responsible for that 'high' feeling in very big doses but in small medicinal doses alongside CBD, it is incredibly effective medicine for helping with symptoms ranging from pain and muscle spasm to sleep and even PTSD symptoms. My patients had been using cannabis as a medicine in various forms themselves for years before I wrote my first prescription for it officially. Often I was the first medical doctor or health professional they had ever discussed it with. The fact that I also had expertise in herbal and botanical medicine as well as conventional made them feel safe enough to tell me about their self-discoveries using cannabis for treating everything from insomnia to severe pain and weaning themselves off opioids where conventional medications had often failed them. It became clear that, in these cases, cannabis, which I had been taught in medical school was a dangerous drug of abuse, when used medicinally (and usually lower THC, higher CBD varieties) was making my patients more resilient and dramatically changing their quality of life. I started to help them navigate how to use it best, minimize side effects and understand the difference between different plant compounds like CBD and THC, and started to speak with my US colleagues who were a few years ahead and already prescribing it for their patients with incredible results. This led to becoming an expert in medicinal cannabis and treating thousands of patients over a number of years, first in Canada and now in the UK. It is still one of the single most powerful tools I have as an integrative medicine and resilience doctor.

The ECS is actually involved in all of the aspects of brain and cell resilience, from protecting your mitochondria and healing the gut, to increasing a brain chemical called BDNF (brain derived neurotropic factor) which helps promote new brain cells and brain flexibility and helps the brain cope better with stress.

The ECS's role in brain resilience is likely one reason why medical cannabis and CBD can work so well for so many diverse symptoms that can seem totally unrelated at first glance. For example, for patients suffering with chronic fatigue syndrome and related conditions like Long Covid, cannabis and even hemp-derived over-the-counter CBD products can make a difference for symptom relief and functioning, especially combined with an integrative approach. Although not a cure, this plant medicine can help with stress and inflammation, pain, mood and sleep. That's because the chemicals called cannabinoids in the cannabis plant work in our ECS, similarly to the natural chemicals we make called 'endocannabinoids'.

Genetic differences in our ECS are now thought to contribute to a greater susceptibility to chronic stress. For example, preliminary research shows that people who carry a certain gene may have a malfunctioning body-chemical receptor in the ECS, called the CB2 receptor. Having this gene means you may have an increased risk of developing depression when exposed to chronic mild stress. This is important for moody types most of all. However, even if you do have these gene, it doesn't mean you are doomed to suffer with low moods and depression for ever. You can still shift these tendencies. But what it does help explain is why you may be more sensitive to stress than someone else. Knowing this sometimes helps remove the feeling of guilt that many people who suffer from chronic mental-health conditions feel. They often feel like 'they should just be tougher' or other people seem to be able to just cope better. But we are all unique and each of us has our own set of challenges and our genes can play a role in our vulnerability to certain health issues, whether it's depression or diabetes. All it means is that we have to be more gentle and forgiving of ourselves in these areas and nurture these aspects of our health more than average.

Gut Health: The Brain–Gut Axis, Leaky Gut and Leaky Brain

There is a saying in integrative medicine: 'When in doubt, start with the gut.' This is in relation to trying to figure out where to start when helping a new patient or client who arrives at the end of their rope, with a long shopping list of diagnoses and medical issues that all seem to overlap. Most of these patients will tell you that they have already 'tried everything'. Starting with the gut is not a new concept. Most traditional medicine systems emphasized the importance of gut health, including the classical Indian system of medicine, Ayurveda, and the Ancient Greeks, who believed many diseases started due to a gut-related imbalance in what they called bile. There was no way of knowing back then the exact biological reasons for this central importance of gut health to overall health, but they had discovered this link of health to the gut by observation over many generations. At last the science is starting to catch up. Restoring gut health is part of the integrative medicine approach to not just getting rid of a bloated belly or irritable bowel (IBS), but seemingly unrelated issues with mood, immunity, energy levels and brain function too. This makes sense because we actually have a little brain in our gut, along with its own nervous system called the enteric nervous system or ENS. It is also rich in receptors for the ECS we just learned about, which explains why my patients with many gut diseases, ranging from Crohn's disease to IBS, respond so well to medical cannabis.

This gut brain, nervous system and gut ECS talks to our 'big brain' in a two-way communication highway. The gut brain also talks to our immune system. Most of our serotonin, one of the main neurotransmitters you can think of as your happy brain chemical (although it is so much more), is actually made in our gut, not our brains. Our gut is quite directly related to mood balance, whether it's helping protect us from anxiety (wound-up warriors) or buffering us against depression (moody warriors).

PSYCHOBIOTICS

Even a decade ago, the idea that beneficial bugs or bacteria (probiotics) could have a direct impact on the brain and mental-health symptoms was pretty radical and quite fringe, almost quacky. However, now this idea is supported by a host of research. Research into the mental-health and brain effects from gut bugs has become a whole field centred around these so-called psychobiotics, or specific types of probiotic strains that influence our gut-bacteria–brain relationships. Psychobiotics can lead to brain changes in areas of emotional, cognitive (thinking), brain-neurochemical balance and brain immune-system function (remember those microglia!), leading to potential anti-anxiety and mood-boosting effects, although it's usually not just as simple as taking a single supplement and completely solving one of these complex issues. We still have a lot to work out because the gut–brain–immune system and bacteria relationships are so complex. Even so, there are some promising early developments. Giving pregnant and postpartum women lactobacillus probiotics to support brain–gut health has been shown to decrease anxiety and depression levels postpartum (after delivery), which in turn has brain benefits for both mums and babies by decreasing stress-hormone negative effects on the brain.[6]

Because the gut–brain–immune-system communication goes both ways, psychological 'bad stress' that affects the brain can also trigger changes in the gut, by potentially altering the healthy gut microbiome, the make-up of different bacteria and yeast which grow and thrive, and shifting the bug community towards less healthy, happy ones. Psychological interventions like cognitive behavioural therapy (CBT), meditation and other stress-coping strategies can actually impact and shift the gut microbiome too. Taking this one step further, when we transplant 'bad bugs' into the gut of healthy animals, they start to exhibit signs of depression, and preliminary research in humans points towards a similar trend: that the billions of tiny microbes in our intestines can actually influence our mood and behaviour in the brain and, ultimately, impact resilience.

Leaky Gut

The brain fog and lack of mental clarity experienced by especially scattered and exhausted warriors when they get out of balance can also relate back to the gut – in this case, a leaky gut. This is when the gut lining starts to become more porous, allowing things like food proteins or toxins to get through intact, setting off an immune response that includes lots of pro-inflammatory cytokines, or immune chemicals which can lead to symptoms of poor stress tolerance and feeling anxious, depressed or constantly fatigued or foggy-headed, depending on your make-up.

Although the research is still really in its infancy in this area, so far it appears that a leaky gut and even a leaky brain barrier can have a direct impact on multiple aspects of resilience.

On the other hand, a healthy microbiome and gut immune system actually helps make the right amounts of the very brain chemicals that keep us resilient: things like GABA (a calming brain chemical that helps buffer brain stress), BDNF (which makes new brain cells so we can learn and remember things), serotonin and many more. A lack of these brain- and body-balancing chemicals due to an unhealthy gut may lead to massive issues in the brain and body, including certain types of 'inflammatory dementia' as well as depression, autoimmune issues and other low-resilience states.

Some integrative medicine clinicians and researchers, including myself, often use advanced functional medicine tests to assess the health of the microbiome, the leakiness of the gut (the gut-lining barrier between the bloodstream and the gut contents) as well as the blood–brain barrier (the brain-lining barrier between the rest of the bloodstream and the brain) when doing an integrative medicine assessment for issues ranging from gut symptoms and women's health issues to depression, fatigue and early memory decline. Once detected, a leaky gut and brain protocol involving foods, supplements and lifestyle changes may help heal these natural barriers and even reverse symptoms that had not responded to conventional therapy thus far, although the science is still in its infancy and again, as is the theme with most integrative medicine areas, there is no single 'quick fix'.

Helping support a healthy gut in the first place may help prevent or at least reduce the severity of these more serious medical issues in those who may be prone to them based on things like their genes. We are discovering how to do this and customize this sort of 'gut-resilience' plan with more precision each day. By using the resilience-medicine toolkit in Part Two of this book, including finding your mind–body practice, diet and supplement tips for your type, you can also help tune up your gut health.

Mitochondrial Factors

Mitochondria are our cell's energy factories. Increasingly, how well those factories are working is being recognized as affecting many aspects of health and resilience. They are the source of our energy in each cell and also involved with programmed cell death which prunes away the bad or dysfunctional cells so that they don't cause an issue. This is literally resilience on a cellular level. Many factors may contribute to our mitochondria not working as well as they could, such as exposure to certain medications (especially if taken over a long period of time) like many antibiotics, statins, certain anti-fungals, acetaminophen (paracetamol) and possibly many more. Other things like mould exposure, nutritional insufficiencies and chronic stress also play a role in how well our little powerhouses make energy.

Mitochondrial dysfunction seems to play a role in diverse chronic diseases, including chronic fatigue, connective tissue diseases (like Ehlers Danlos where people are also hyperflexible as well) and so many others. How much something impacts our energy factories seems to vary quite widely from person to person. Like most things with human beings, our genes likely play a role too in how sensitive we are to these things. In general, I have found exhausted warriors tend to be most sensitive to signs of mitochondrial dysfunction. There is no single blood test to check optimal mitochondrial function, although some functional medicine tests such as organic acids panels may give an indirect measure. However, the most important thing for now, until we have more direct testing, is to minimize things that can zap your mitochondria and max out the things that are good for them. For example, a resilience diet, specific supplements, and having a stress-reducing mind–body practice all make your mitochondria quite happy (see Part Two of this book). Then there are things like alcohol and some recreational substances such as cocaine and methamphetamine, which also damage our mitochondria and impair their ability to function properly, so are best to minimize or avoid completely if you have chronically low energy.

A note on alcohol: Part of my work is in harm reduction and drug policy reform. When people ask me about the harm factor of certain substances, they are always quite shocked to hear that, from a health perspective, alcohol is at the top of the list in terms of addictive potential, risk to resilience and health compared with other classes of substances such as the psychedelic drugs including LSD. These have a much lower harm ratio generally, are non-addictive and do not seem to impair mitochondrial function. Alcohol, on the other hand, is a mitochondrial poison. One of the cheapest, quickest* and first interventions I do with any of my patients who have chronic fatigue or brain fog is to cut out alcohol completely and substitute it for an alcohol-free spirit (see food chapter in Part Two) for socializing. Sometimes we add a cannabis medicine if they were using alcohol to self-medicate their anxiety, stress, mood or pain condition. At the same time, more people are choosing not to drink alcohol or do so only occasionally for lifestyle reasons even if they don't have a medical condition. These societal shifts may lead to improved resilience on a population level over time due to the impact on our mitochondria, brain and body.

BDNF – the Brain's Secret Resilience Factor

Another factor that helps regulate and rein in the limbic system and the HPA axis in the face of chronic stress is the brain chemical called BDNF (brain derived neurotrophic factor). This is a key brain chemical that actually helps the brain learn how to turn off the maladaptive chronic stress response. Basically, the more BDNF your brain makes in the right parts of the brain, the better you are at adapting to stress, the lower your allosteric load (which is the technical term for the total brain-and-body stress burden) and the higher your resilience becomes. Like all resilience factors, how much BDNF we make is a combination of our genes plus our environment and life experiences, but luckily there are proven ways to boost it.

It has been shown that everything from diet (binning the western diet of highly processed 'bad fats' combined with high amounts of refined sugar and replacing it with what I call the 'resilience diet' which you will learn about next in Part Two) to exercise, optimal sleep and even changing our environment can enhance the brain's

---

* Note: For people who may be suffering from alcohol addiction or dependency, a formal medical detox and rehab programme is needed for safety. If you are concerned you may have an addiction or dependency issue, always seek professional help.

ability to make more Brain Derived Neurotophic Factor (BDNF). Plant medicines and psychedelics may also enhance BDNF.

So this means you can start turning what might currently feel like overwhelming 'bad stress' into more of that 'good stress' over time without quitting your job and living in a cave (thank goodness!). Most of the people I meet who come to me for help with stress, resilience and related issues actually don't want to 'check out' from their life: there's lots of good in there too, but they can't carry on as they are without a major stress reset so that they can cope better in daily life and have more joy with less pressure.

NPY

NPY, or neuropeptide Y, is another brain resilience peptide, or protein, and biomarker that is becoming more researched for its wide-ranging effects on mood, appetite, stress, circadian rhythms, alcohol addiction and PTSD.

Higher amounts of NYP are linked to higher resilience and its job appears to involve dampening down sympathetic nervous system overactivity in the face of stress so that it doesn't reach toxic levels. People with PTSD and depression have lower NPY levels, but when treated with an antidepressant drug called escitalopram, their NPY levels started to increase and normalize again.[7] This is a great example of why, as part of resilience medicine, combining drugs and natural approaches can be effective in certain situations.

Galanin

Galanin is another brain protein important for resilience. It has a role, like NPY, in modulating our fight-or-flight response to stress, and is neuroprotective and promotes neurogenesis (e.g. improves brain flexibility) too. There is a lot of this protein in brain areas such as the *locus coeruleus*, which is involved in the stress response. It acts there as a counterbalance, helping dampen down the activation of this brain-stress area so that stress doesn't become the toxic, bad kind.

In animals, physical exercise increases brain galanin levels, which is likely one of the very many reasons why exercise can enhance resilience for every type, especially when you find the best type for you (see Part Two).

The Magic of Synergy

What so much of this recent research has taught us is that what are categorized as mental illnesses have a biological basis, even when it's hard to see or measure. This is contrary to what doctors believed until quite recently. And conversely, psychological therapies can also help to change biomarkers, or biology and physical symptoms, in a bi-directional system. This is why resilience medicine includes both biological (e.g. food, supplements, power plants like CBD and medical cannabis, some medications) and mind–body interventions to help create a more resilient brain and body over time. If you already suffer from symptoms or a chronic condition, it can help improve these, but even if you don't, a synergetic approach can help decrease your chances of developing an issue down the road by helping you become more resilient to bad stress at a brain, body and cellular level.

The individual combination of resilience factors each of us is born with and can alter over the course of our life, based on our environment and experiences, is endless. Our resilience level is affected by every brain-chemical system, ranging from our reward system (involving dopamine, which may be especially important if you are a scattered type) to our happiness and mood system (via serotonin, especially important to wound-up and moody warriors).

It's impossible to tease each of these factors apart and isolate them because they all affect each other. However, the good news is that by introducing a set of resilience habits and small changes, you can impact many of these systems simultaneously to help bring more balance to your life and supercharge your resilience powers. That is what we will do in Part Two, using the resilience toolkit to help you on your resilience journey.

Resilient Hormones

There's a lot of talk about 'hormone balancing' in the mainstream media these days, but what exactly is a hormone? It's a chemical that sends specific messages throughout the brain and body and many hormones are needed in the right combinations for a resilient brain and body. Hormones are important for everyone, but the most common reasons people come to see me for 'hormone help' are related to women's health issues in different life phases. For example, problems like nightmare periods or more serious issues like endometriosis and PCOS, suboptimal fertility and, a bit later on, for perimenopausal and then menopausal/post-menopausal issues related to hormone health. However, men also need a balance of healthy hormones too, although men's hormone health is less publicized. Hormones in both men and women also play a role in issues related to the thyroid, which affects energy levels, and also issues related to that HPA stress axis, causing low stress tolerance. There are many hormones which are important and they all tend to work together in the brain and body, but I'll just focus on some of the most important ones and what they do in a nutshell to impact resilience (and what you can do to help them!).

Stress Hormones

The hormones of the HPA axis are central to resilience. CRH is the first hormone in the HPA-axis stress-response pathway we learned about earlier. Differences in the genes for the CRH receptor appear to influence how likely someone is to experience more anxiety under stress (hello, wound-up warriors!).

Cortisol, the next hormone in the HPA-axis pathway, is one of the best-known steroid hormones and is made by the adrenal glands. It is needed to help you in acutely stressful scenarios, but as we learned, it becomes toxic to brain cells, especially those in the hippocampus involved in memory and learning, if it hangs around all of the time in high amounts, i.e. becomes chronically high. As part of an integrative medicine approach, we can measure the amount of cortisol in the saliva at different times of day, starting in the very early morning until late at night, to create a pattern over twenty-four hours, or a circadian-rhythm pattern for this hormone. This pattern tells us if cortisol is peaking and falling at the wrong time of day, in which case it can lead to the 'tired-yet-wired' issue experienced by so many people, especially exhausted warriors. If this is an issue for you, there are things we can do, from sleep hygiene and sleeping in complete darkness to taking supplements to help restore the balance. (You will find more on sleep in Part Two.)

DHEA is another steroid hormone that helps enhance resilience and it has been shown in studies that having a low DHEA:cortisol ratio (meaning you do not have enough DHEA) is associated with low-resilience states such as chronic fatigue syndrome, anxiety, PTSD, depression and burnout. Conversely, in a group of healthy men, being given a DHEA supplement improved memory and mood. Managing bad stress can help keep the ratio of DHEA to cortisol optimal, via a resilience programme including mind–body practices, foods and adding herbal adaptogens (see Part Two). Sometimes, in menopause and andropause (the hormone change experienced in later life in men), DHEA applied through the skin may be part of an integrative medicine treatment approach to help reduce symptoms (under a doctor's supervision), but it is not recommended for everyone.

Thyroid Hormones

The thyroid gland in the neck controls metabolic rate, some aspects of digestion and bone health. A suboptimal thyroid gland can also affect your sleep, mental sharpness, energy levels and how easily you gain fat weight, and can make you more sensitive to hot and cold as it also controls temperature regulation and many immune-system functions. The thyroid is also controlled by the brain in the hypothalamus, by the HPT axis which stands for the hypothalamic–pituitary–thyroid axis. You can think of it as the sister to the HPA axis, which controls the adrenal glands and cortisol hormone. These two systems also talk to each other, influence each other and both need to be working well for tip-top resilience. The first hormone to check to make sure your thyroid is working well is called thyroid stimulating hormone, or TSH. However, for some people with more subtle thyroid issues, the TSH can remain in the broad so-called 'normal' range while the actual functioning is below optimal, causing issues like fatigue, difficulty losing weight and intolerance to cold. As an integrative medicine doctor, I check not just TSH but also the other thyroid hormones: Free T3, Free T4 and Reverse T3. If there are issues in any of these hormones, it can signal a hormone imbalance in this system which we then address using an integrative approach with botanicals, supplements, dietary measures and, when necessary, medication. Fixing a suboptimal thyroid issue can have a huge positive impact on resilience, especially if you suffer with unexplained fatigue and haven't had this checked.

Women's Health Hormones: Oestrogens and Progesterone and the HPO axis

Just as the brain's hypothalamus tells the adrenal glands what to do with cortisol and the thyroid gland what to do with its hormones (T3, T4 and reverse T3), it also instructs the ovaries in women. This pathway is called the HPO or hypothalamic–pituitary–ovarian axis. The brain releases two hormones, FSH and LH, which control the ovaries and the menstrual cycles. The ovaries then produce oestrogen and progesterone as well as small amounts of testosterone. If the oestrogen:progesterone ratio is off, you get issues. Too much estrogen, an issue called oestrogen dominance, it is associated with anxiety before your period and also more serious issues like endometriosis (a painful condition where womb tissue grows outside the womb), polycystic ovarian syndrome (PCOS) and fertility issues. On the other hand, if oestrogen is too low relative to progesterone, it is associated more with depression or 'moody PMS'. We need oestrogen in the right forms (there are three different ones: 2-hydroxyestrone, 16-hydroxyestrone and 4-hydroxyestrone) and in the right amount because it has 400 crucial functions in the brain and body, ranging from helping with brain and memory function to regulating blood sugar (oestrogen improves insulin sensitivity so it's anti-diabetic) and helping with heart health. It also enhances energy and mood when in the right balance. Oestrogen and progesterone balance also plays a role in mental clarity and cognition. During the perimenopause, brain fog and poor memory are thought to be caused, in part, by this shift in hormones and lower amounts of oestrogen.

Sharron came to see me for 'menopause'. However, when we dug down into what was bothering her the most, it wasn't hot flushes. It was the brain fog, fatigue and 'over-the-top' anxiety, feeling constantly stressed and irritable most days since 'the transition'. She was still getting some periods, so technically she was in perimenopause. I explained to her that her changing up and down hormone levels, combined with oestrogen not being there in the same amounts to help her counter the stress response in the brain, was likely a big contributing cause of her symptoms. She had always been 'uptight' and a bit anxious before perimenopause, but it was manageable. That is often the case especially for wound-up warriors when they hit perimenopause. Their 'off switch' combined with the fluctuating hormone levels leads to stress overwhelm.

Sharron waited so long to see a doctor because she had been told by a friend that HRT was dangerous and high risk for causing cancer and she didn't think there was 'much else' she could do besides 'get more sleep and eat healthily'. I explained that for most women, including her, body-identical HRT in the lowest dose needed to control her symptoms was low risk. She decided to start this and we combined it with a high CBD oil to help with stress and a very low dose of THC-containing medical cannabis oil at night to help her sleep, since sleeping pills had given her unwanted side effects and her poor sleep was making her feel foggy during the day. I gave her a relaxing breathing exercise to do a few minutes a day and we added a few supplements for stress support. We also tested her thyroid to make sure it was working optimally. In three months, she was back to her 'old self' again but 'better' and felt more relaxed and in control of her stress levels than she had in years.

Women's hormones are connected to resilience and our stress and energy hormone systems too. So when I see someone who has come in for help with anxiety, again more common in wound-up warriors,

I always ask about their cycles and often find they are also having trouble here. The same goes for moody warriors, I always investigate how hormones may be playing a role in their mood ups and downs. We have to balance all of these three pathways to get brain resilience back on track.

Testosterone

Both men and women make testosterone (T) in the adrenal glands and men also make more in the testes whereas women make some small amounts in the ovaries. In men and women, this is also a resilience hormone because healthy T levels support brain-cell survival. It has been found that men who have very low testosterone are at increased risk of developing dementia in later life. In women, testosterone can't work properly in the brain without enough oestrogen to help it out. That is why if body identical HRT is considered, sometimes a small amount of testosterone is added to the oestrogen and progesterone therapy, something that can bring a tremendous amount of relief to many women especially when added to botanicals, medical cannabis and mind–body approaches for more severe perimenopausal symptoms.

Oxytocin

Oxytocin is often called the snuggle hormone. It has a number of important jobs in the brain related to resilience, including social and emotional processing and social bonding, pain processing and empathy. Some studies have shown, for example, that people who suffered emotional trauma or PTSD have lower levels of oxytocin. In dads with postpartum depression, treatment with an oxytocin nasal spray increased the activation of brain circuits involved in reward, empathy and attention towards their toddlers.[8] Oxytocin is likely an adaptive hormone to help with successful social bonding, an aspect of social intelligence. And the great news is we can get more oxytocin simply by giving a loved one a hug and having an element of supportive physical intimacy, sharing close space with others in a purely platonic or non-romantic way where we feel safe and supported.

The Biology of a 'Resilience Temperament'

Researchers have also noticed that there are certain temperamental traits which seem to be associated with resilience and allow people to bounce back incredibly even after experiencing severe trauma. No matter where you are right now on the resilience spectrum, all the brain, immune-system, gut and cell factors described can also be boosted by cultivating what is known as a 'resilience temperament'. Even if you are not born with natural resilience, these resilience traits are learnable skills. Many mind–body practices and mental habits can help us hone different aspects of these resilient traits. It has been demonstrated that several of these traits overlap with a higher EQ, or emotional intelligence, which has been shown to enhance resilience because these traits can help turn threats into challenges. EQ and resilience traits are a skill set we can all enhance, regardless of our personality, how outgoing we are or any health problems we may be suffering with.

Even small, simple mental shifts can help us adopt more of these traits over time, no matter what our resilience type is. Each type may be prone to difficulty in one or more of these traits. For example, wound-up warriors may find their challenge is building self-confidence and not worrying about pleasing people whereas moody warriors can struggle with self-empathy and seeing things as glass half-full, or optimism. Scattered types may struggle with self-awareness and reading other people, and exhausted warriors can struggle with their 'get up and go' or, as I like to call it, their innate life energy and passion factor, often due to a lack of energy resources. All types when unbalanced can become rigid and less tolerant, so this is universally something to work on, no matter what your type.

Top-ten Resilience Temperament Traits

Compassion

Empathy is the ability to understand and share what someone else is feeling. Compassion goes one step further. It's being able to understand someone's struggles and empathize without 'getting down into the hole' with them. This is key for resilience because being overly empathetic can be draining if you start feeling the same strong negative/sad/mad emotions as someone you are empathizing with, even though it may help them feel better. It is also different from sympathy, which is about 'feeling bad' for someone or even pity and, again, becoming sad yourself or trying to give advice to reduce your own feelings of discomfort. Both sympathy and empathy when they're overdone can lead to feeling distressed in response to other people's distress. Whereas compassion makes you feel warm and fuzzy, genuinely concerned for the other person but without the distress. Compassion also activates your brain's reward networks. Feeling compassion makes a different part of your brain light up than the parts associated with sympathy or even empathy.[9]

Scattered types tend to struggle with cultivating compassion and also empathy for others, whereas exhausted warriors tend to be overly empathetic and sympathetic, which leads to burnout. However, everyone can enhance their compassion quotient to lead to adaptive interactions and all the benefits of empathy without the energy drain. Practising active listening, acknowledging other people's feelings if they appear sad or upset, paying attention to others body language for cues on how they are feeling and doing your best to giving advice and simply listen instead of trying to 'fix' are all ways to build compassion.

Compassion meditation styles are probably the most direct and simplest way to help enhance this skill over time (see Part Two). There are also many therapy schools of thought that teach compassion training as a skill, such as one called Internal Family Systems among others. This is an especially good skill for moody types, who tend to struggle with self-compassion specifically. It turns out having compassion for yourself also helps you have more compassion and empathy for other people too.

Optimism

Optimists see the world through a glass-half-full filter. Glass-half-full thinkers are experts in finding the so-called silver lining in what may initially feel like a threatening or negative situation. This ability to find even a kernel of good or to cultivate a positive emotional feeling in the face of extreme challenge is a huge determining factor in how your brain perceives your experience. Two people could experience exactly the same event but perceive it completely differently, depending on their levels of optimism. For tips on how to become more of an optimist, see the suggestions for moody warriors in the mind–body chapter in Part Two (page 181).

Self-awareness

This skill has to do with being aware of and able to assess your own emotions, bringing these emotional experiences to the conscious level where you can process and then release them. This means your emotions don't get boxed off and take up mental space. Developing self-awareness can help if you tend to feel overwhelmed by strong emotions. Keeping a journal of emotional events as well as a mindfulness-based naming-emotions practice are two evidence-based ways to enhance this trait (see Part Two under mind–body for details on how to do them). Being 'hyper'-aware, however, can also become counterproductive if it leads to excessive worrying and rumination, which can be a tendency of a wound-up warrior. Hyper-awareness can also overlap with people pleasing and social anxiety. When self-awareness is coupled with the next resilience trait, self-regulation, it can rein in these tendencies and avoid these mental traps.

Self-regulation

The skill of self-regulation is closely linked with self-awareness. It is the ability, after you have become aware of your emotions, to then act in a way that is most consistent with resilience. For example, avoiding knee-jerk responses and reducing stress reactivity when under pressure. That means, if you have a temper, learning to express anger safely and to release it rather than letting it boil over into snappiness or aggression. Self-regulation is also related to the ability to self-soothe and regulation of the autonomic nervous system like we learned about earlier.

Self-regulation is a skill we start developing in infancy and childhood and is tied to the skill of being able to self-calm at an early age in response to a stressor or frustration. Learning this early ability to self-calm helps us become better able to handle stress and frustration as we get older and become adults. Not everyone has ideal conditions in childhood to learn these skills, but luckily we can enhance this trait as adults. It just takes time and patience. Practising mindfulness daily (see Part Two) can help us avoid knee-jerk responses by giving our brains a mental pause. Working with a professional psychotherapist on self-soothing skills or using a self-care app to help us in claiming responsibility for our own emotions/actions and pausing between emotion and action can also develop this skill further. Other practices like HRV training (see Part Two, in the mind–body chapter, page 181) using an inexpensive heart-rate monitoring device may also enhance our nervous system's ability to self-regulate better over time.

High Self-esteem

Increasing self-esteem, self-belief and self-confidence has been shown to enhance resilience and decrease vulnerability in multiple studies on addictions, depression and social stressors.[10,11,12] Often someone may appear quite confident but in reality lack a deeper self-esteem and still be prone to more stressful reactions to perceived failure. Sometimes this lack of self-confidence can ironically come off as arrogance.

Deeper self-esteem involves a reframing of perceived failures and a willingness to try again. It also involves the attitude that you always can learn something from other people. Many of the most expert people I know within their chosen fields still have a beginner's mentality when it comes to being open to a new idea or concept that could shift the way they do things, even within their own areas of expertise, which is also linked to the trait of being flexible. These attitudes ultimately lead to more successes over time, which further builds self-esteem and confidence. Self-esteem and self-confidence at this deeper level buffer us from mental distress, which in turn changes the stress reaction in the brain. Building self-esteem is a process, but doing something as simple and enjoyable as listening to empowering music can help boost it, according to research.[13] 'Reframing' techniques such as CBT (cognitive behavioural therapy) which includes challenging negative self-beliefs and interrupting negative self-talk can help too. Something called narrative therapy, which helps people to be the narrator of their own life story and regain that sense of self-empowerment that may be lacking, is another tool to improve this skill if you don't necessarily jive with traditional CBT.

Socially Connected

By socially connected, I mean someone who is highly competent at interpersonal relationships. This skill set is all about enhancing our relationships with others and strengthening our social bonds. It's the ability to connect with others of varying personality types and in many different situations. Different types can have different challenges in this area when out of balance: wound-up warriors can get social anxiety, moodys can tend to isolate themselves, exhausted types tend to overextend their energies and then burn themselves out and scattereds have a hard time remembering important events or keeping in touch.

Making small changes such as really listening to others' stories without interrupting, and resisting the urge to fill every gap with talking to relieve anxiety can help you connect better with others, as well as give someone genuine praise. When we become more sensitive to the emotional needs of other people, they are more likely to want to engage with us, offer help and assistance and reciprocate that emotional support. This leads to stronger social relationships and a web of support that helps with our bounce-back factor when bad or challenging things happen. The effect of social connection on health and resilience has become a 'hot topic' in mainstream medicine. Lots of research has been done looking at the 'Science of Connection'. And what they have found is pretty amazing. Social connection can actually change our biology of resilience and is not just 'fluff'. A healthy social network and warm close relationships shape resilience, as has been proven in multiple large studies. In other research, it has been shown that being well integrated socially reduces all-cause age-adjusted mortality by a factor of two – about as much as having low versus high serum cholesterol levels or being a non-smoker.

Passionate Zest

This is the trait related to what I call having an innate life energy or 'zest' for life. Having an element of passion and just plain old fun in your life also aids resilience, whether it is for a specific hobby, your work, looking after family or anything that brings you joy and fulfilment. Having fun can bring a sense of light-heartedness that helps reduce stress and strain in everyday life. It doesn't have to involve a fancy vacation or spending money. Injecting more fun and joy into everyday life can be as simple as watching a funny movie, or using humour to defuse stressful situations. Some people find a more formal practice like laughter yoga can really help, or scheduling some fun time into the diary so you can bring more conscious attention to this human need and desire. If this is something you are currently lacking, fear not. It is never too late to start activating this 'joie de vivre'. In one study on burnout and emotional exhaustion in healthcare workers, having more fun at work was found to be a protective, or resilience, factor against burnout. Having fun is now also considered to be integral to workplace performance too and the best hundred companies in *Fortune* magazine all have a 'fun factor' in their workplace culture. Fun isn't the only aspect of passion, however. Passionate zest is also related to feeling like your life has purpose and meaning, another factor which helps get us through bad times and challenges with greater ease and less suffering.

Self-motivation

This trait is about being able to take initiative or be a self-starter. It also involves generating drive towards achievement, commitment to a project or cause, and seeing things through. This trait can be a challenging one, especially important for moody types and also some scattered types who struggle to focus. But it's really important because not being able to really visualize your dreams and goals and then execute the necessary steps towards them can make you feel impotent in creating the life you truly want. A lack of self-motivation can also hinder self-belief and a loss of a sense of purpose, two other resilience traits. The good news is that you can work on self-motivation as a skill even if it's not your strong suit. Goal setting using what are known as 'SMART' goals (Specific, Measurable, Achievable, Relevant, and Time-bound) and writing them out once a season can help. Also helpful is (whenever possible) to pick projects that excite you or bring you joy, and when you are not loving a particular project, try to find at least one good thing that might help you to keep going and find satisfaction in that work.

Tolerance

Resilient temperaments are also more tolerant ones. They tend not to hold grudges and are more understanding of others' shortcomings and of their own limitations. The opposite of this is setting impossible standards for everyone, leading to frustration and disappointment, something wound-up warriors tend to be most prone to. One reason tolerance breeds resilience may relate back to having the capacity for more compassion for yourself and others when you can adopt a more forgiving attitude. It also helps rein in perfectionism, which can be a toxic mix when combined with stress and affect other resilience traits like self-esteem, flexibility and self-regulation.

Flexibility

Resilient people are more flexible in terms of their thinking, not how easily they can touch their toes. As we learned, brain flexibility is central to resilience and involves adapting those brain networks and shifting states in response to stress and unexpected curveballs. People who can be more flexible and adapt to change more easily feel less of the bad sort of stress on a brain level. Flexible thinking also leads to creative ways of solving problems that if approached in a rigid way may appear unsolvable at first glance. Plans change at the last minute or the unexpected happens? Flexible people are able to adapt quickly without getting angry or upset about the changes, whether it's a flight that got delayed or the place you planned to meet up with a friend. This can relate to relationship or interpersonal problems, or to health challenges, in terms of seeing things in a new light in order to come up with a solution that may not have previously been considered.

Even if you cultivate and enhance just one of these ten resilience traits over time, the changes will then start to impact multiple biological resilience factors in the brain and in your body cells in a positive feedback loop. Our thoughts and beliefs are powerful drivers of our biology, as I hope I have convinced you by the end of this chapter.

Many people may seem, from the outside at least, 'naturally' gifted with a resilient temperament, which seems a bit unfair. However, if you feel you are not naturally adept at many of these resilience traits, don't worry because they are also learnable skills and not just reserved for a lucky few. Depending on your resilience type, building some of these skills may be more challenging for you than others and that's OK too. Now that we have a clearer sense of the science of resilience, in Part Two we will look at ways of building these traits as actionable skills and also using foods, supplements and power plants to help enhance our resilience biology.

Part Two

The Resilience Toolkit

CHAPTER THREE

THE CIRCADIAN RHYTHM RESET

'Sleep is the best meditation'
Dalai Lama

When I asked my patient Mary how she slept, her response was 'Fine.'
She reported going to bed before midnight, getting up at the same time
each day after making sure she got seven and a half hours most nights
and she even proudly told me that she avoided coffee after dinner.
However, she was coming to see me for chronic low energy and more
frequent flare-ups of her autoimmune disease. In these situations,
experience tells me that, even when a patient says their sleep is fine, it
should still be one of the first places we start. Mary was an exhausted
warrior and when we dug deeper into her sleep quality, it was clear
things weren't as fine as she thought: it took her thirty minutes or more
to fall asleep and she reported being a very light sleeper, waking multiple
times a night. Most mornings she felt groggy and unrested, despite being
in bed for seven and a half hours with her eyes closed. This pattern had
been the same for so many years, she didn't know anything else and so
this had just become normal for her. Insomnia, she thought, meant people
who were up 'all night' staring at the wall, so her more subtle signs of
sleep dysfunction 'didn't really count'. She was also shocked that no doctor before had ever connected any of her symptoms with her poor sleep
quality and that improving her sleep could have an effect on seemingly
unrelated symptoms and autoimmune disease activity.

Resetting Sleep

When I talk about sleep, I'm not just concerned about the hours you spend in bed. That is because how well we rest at night is a barometer of twenty-four-hour circadian-rhythm health. What that means is that our brains and bodies are programmed to do certain things and make specific amounts of chemicals, hormones and neurotransmitters at different times a day. We make melatonin, our sleep hormone, at night and serotonin, our happy hormone, during the day (this is a bit of an oversimplification but you get the idea). Our stress hormones peak in the morning to wake us up and wind down to allow us to fall asleep without leaving us feeling 'jacked'. When sleep is out of whack, so are these hormone cycles – which can wreak havoc on everything from mood and focus to stress levels and immune-system health.

HOW MY HUSBAND FIXED MY LIGHT SLEEPING

During medical school I had been completely sensitized to my pager going off in the middle of the night and had since become a very light sleeper. Nick, my boyfriend at the time (now husband) was a clinical hypnotherapist and had also studied yoga nidra in India. He started doing live relaxation-training-guided yoga nidra meditations for me before sleep every night.

I was stubborn and sceptical but he made it so easy and calming that I stuck with it. The first thing I noticed was that I fell asleep so much quicker! Then, as the weeks went on, I was less hypersensitive to sounds and slept more deeply. It took time and patience because my brain was on hyper-alert and being on call kept it alert – I needed lots of time and regular practice to get my brain to 'reboot' in the face of my nervous system's hyper-arousal. This is typical of wound-up warriors when out of balance. The better I slept, the more energy I had during the day, the quicker I got over colds and the sharper I felt.

Although I still wear earplugs to sleep since my sleep is more sensitive than average (genetics play a role in this too), yoga nidra made a huge difference and it is a practice I still come back to till this day if I am feeling stressed and sleeping poorly, or if I'm in a less-than-optimal sleep environment – for example, while travelling or on an overnight flight. I also sometimes combine it with a small amount of medicinal cannabis and sleepy herbs which is even more effective than yoga nidra alone.

You can find yoga nidra recordings online either in wellbeing and resilience apps (we have developed one at LondonResilience.com that is free to use) or on YouTube.

Before we get started on the sleep reset protocol itself, it's important to understand a bit about why sleep is so critical for resilience. In fact, it is the grounding for the entire resilience programme, no matter what your type. Some types are more prone to different sleep issues. For example, wound-up warriors typically have the most trouble falling asleep, followed by moody warriors. Fragmented, non-restorative sleep is most common and severe with exhausted warriors, but can also be an issue for moody types to a lesser extent, especially waking up in the early morning. Scattered types have the most trouble sticking to a sleep/wake routine and are the most likely to stay up late on screens watching movies or on their phones, which leads to disrupting the brain and body's twenty-four-hour clock and feeling unfocused the next day.

Without working on sleep, the brain will be resistant to change and have fewer mental and physical resources to help you break the core patterns for each resilience type. For example, just one poor night of sleep affects all four resilience types differently:

- Moody: a lack of high-quality sleep makes it harder to regulate your emotions, worsens depression and can even cause it.

Lack of good sleep also causes the brain to interpret your environment in a more negative, even threatening, light.

- Wound-up: poor sleep worsens anxiety and causes brain 'wind-up' or overarousal. This increases the fight-or-flight brain networks and increases stress-hormone levels – the last thing a wound-up warrior needs.
- Scattered: just one night's poor sleep impairs memory and focus to a similar level as if you were drunk. This impairs the ability to ignore distractions to focus on a task, which is bad news if you are already struggling with attention.
- Exhausted: a lack of high-quality sleep worsens fatigue and daytime exhaustion, leading to a vicious cycle of relying on caffeine during the day and substances like alcohol or sleeping pills to relax at night. All of which further disrupt healthy sleep patterns and worsen the problem long term.

It's important to recognize that lack of sleep isn't a night-time problem, but a twenty-four-hour problem. Poor sleep affects multiple specific areas of brain function not just at night but when you are awake too. When we don't sleep well, it leads to chronic nervous-system 'hyper-arousal', keeping us unable to wind back down properly. Relaxation and good sleep is how the brain recovers or bounces back, so you can see that our resilience is highly influenced by how well rested we are. Chronic poor sleep and insomnia is associated with a twenty-four-hour increase of corticotropin and cortisol secretion (stress hormones), increased inflammatory markers and disrupted brain-calming chemicals (such as a neurotransmitter called GABA). Insomnia is also associated with other brain issues such as HPA-axis dysfunction, the stress-regulation system, with cortisol peaking at the wrong time of day making it harder to go to sleep easily and also harder to wake up and feel energized in the mornings. Another brain network called the RAS (reticular activating system), which is in charge of wakefulness but should become quiet during sleep, can become hypervigilant at the wrong time (e.g. at night-time, when you are trying to sleep). This RAS dysfunction is associated with many chronic health conditions including ADD, depression and dementia just to name a few. Other brain areas such as the thalamus, whose job it is to regulate how much stimulation the brain responds to – like a pacemaker for the brain – are also affected by poor sleep, as is the *locus coeruleus*, which is in charge of our sleep/wake switch. So you can see that sleep affects so many areas of the brain, and when our sleep is out of whack, so is everything else!

Now let's look at some specific sleep disruptors and how to handle them. These tips are applicable to all resilience types, but some will be more affected than others.

The LAN Problem and Blue Light

LAN, or Light at Night, is a new phenomenon in recent human history. LAN refers to artificial light (i.e. not sunlight) which, until the end of the nineteenth century was limited to candles and gas lights. Since the industrial revolution, we have shifted to electric lighting. This invention was a major shift in human life both at work and home. It made it possible to work twenty-four hours a day in factories and this meant the first 'night shifts' on a mass scale. It also changed the amount of light we have at home and when we go out socially after dark. Even more significant was that electric light bulbs emit more blue light than candles or gas lamps did. Now we have LED and fluorescent bulbs, which emit even *more* blue light than the old incandescent light bulbs many of us grew up with.

These two major shifts in modern life – having electric bright lights after sunset in our life *and* those lights emitting more blue wavelengths of light – have been a *huge* change for our brains and bodies to adapt to, and in fact, we still haven't adapted.

UV light, and especially light in the blue wavelengths, affects our circadian rhythms, or our daily 'biological clock'. We have special genes called clock genes that control our physiology (for example, hormone levels, inflammation) and even our behaviour to a huge extent. This is a new frontier in medicine, much like our endocannabinoid system or ECS, another system we didn't know about until a few decades ago. Too much LAN and especially blue light after sunset disrupts this all-important rhythm and has been linked in research studies to problems ranging from depression, chronic fatigue, susceptibility to infections and immune-system problems, early dementia and premature ageing to obesity, certain cancers and even diabetes.[1]

But clock genes go even further than this. Based on recent research in animals and some preliminary studies in humans, disruption of the clock genes and our biological clock have direct effects on every resilience type.

For wound-up warriors, clock genes regulate the stress-hormone response, cortisol, and when they get messed up, your stress-hormone levels can peak at the wrong time of the day – at night when you are trying to drift off to sleep – causing the 'jacked-up', nervous-system effect. This can lead to problems falling asleep.

For moody warriors, clock genes also control mood balance, and the ability to maintain an even, positive mood seems to be related to this system. Moody warriors tend to wake up very early in the morning when they get out of balance and can't fall back to sleep again. This pattern is linked to the brain-fog and thinking issues (called cognitive symptoms) of depression.

Important for all types, but especially exhausted warriors, our clock genes seem to influence our gut microbiome and our immune response to all types of threats, ranging from viral and bacterial infections to autoimmune reactions where the immune system starts attacking itself. Some infections may also directly disrupt our clock genes, leading to further sleep issues and daytime fatigue. Clock genes and the chemicals and cells they influence also seem to control how leaky our blood–brain barrier is. A 'leaky brain' is now suspected to be part of the problem in a host of autoimmune diseases such as multiple sclerosis. It may also play a role in more poorly understood diseases of the immune and nervous system such as fibromyalgia, chronic Lyme and chronic fatigue syndrome or ME. Exhausted warriors tend to have a sleep-disruption pattern when they get out of balance that involves light, fragmented sleep with multiple wake-ups or near wake-ups overnight and needing more total sleep time than average to feel rested (e.g. nine or more hours versus seven and a half per night).

Scattered warriors tend to be more nighthawks than the other types. This can lead to often staying up late on screens and sleeping in later in the mornings, if they are lucky enough to sleep in. If they have to wake up for work, this can lead to feeling pretty awful in the morning but better as the day goes on, due to a shift in the biological clock. This may become even more pronounced when nighthawks use that late-night awake time to take in more damaging blue light from computer and TV screens and smartphones, which turns off the sleep hormone, melatonin, and wakes the brain up.

To recap, LAN is a relatively new phenomenon in terms of human evolution. Now, instead of the brain winding down after the sun sets, in front of a fire or candlelight which is red (safe!) light, our brains start to wind *up* at night in front of blue-light-emitting lights and screens. This blue light tells our brain to be awake and messes up our clock genes, disrupts our sleep/wake cycles, and turns down production of our sleep hormone, melatonin. When we suppress melatonin and disrupt our clock genes, it can lead to a pro-inflammatory, dysregulated brain and body state and impact all aspects of resilience.

How to Reduce LAN and Blue Light Sources in the Evenings

Part of the sleep reset is taking steps to reduce how much blue light our brains are exposed to after sunset, especially in the two or three hours before bedtime. This is obviously easier said than done, since most evening entertainment, especially at home, revolves around a screen of some sort. However, especially if you are suffering with non-restorative sleep or feeling tired during the day without caffeine, it is a necessary step to some degree.

I recommend that for the next two weeks, you have what I call a total 'screen holiday' after 7.30 p.m.

I know that may sound extreme and you may wonder what the heck you are supposed to do to fill all of that time.

Having worked through this with many patients, some ideas that have proven effective are:

- Reading a book (a real one, not on an e-reader with a back light!). I try to pick up books at our local charity bookstore for around a pound a piece and then swap them with friends and family to avoid the inevitable storage issue of a pile-up.
- Catch up with a friend or family member (in person if you can, or if not, block time for audio-call catch-ups so you are not looking at a screen).
- Learn chess, or if that's too much effort, try draughts instead.
- Listen to music, and connect a smart voice-activated speaker so you don't have to look at your phone screen while you find what you like.
- Do some home yoga or other gentle movement exercise on the ground, or some gentle stretching.
- Go for a walk after dinner.
- Play a board game.

In my medical practice, when I am treating someone whose resilience is on the very low end of the spectrum, we sometimes extend this no screens after 7.30 p.m. rule to eight weeks and then slowly, using blue-blocking glasses (see below), allow a small window of screens in the evening, but still none after 8.30 p.m. This is a major change to life, but because the alterations to the clock genes can take months to right themselves and the changes take time to kick in, especially if you are suffering from a more long-standing condition such as depression, chronic fatigue syndrome, burnout or an autoimmune issue, the longer you can stick to this the better it will work.

In addition, my advice for all resilience types, even if you don't think you have particularly bad sleep issues, is to take your blue-light exposure seriously. I'd advise all types to follow this advice:

- Turn off *all screens*, including smart phones, and set devices to airplane mode in the bedroom so they don't light up overnight while you sleep.

- *No* flashing blinking lights for charging cables in the bedroom.
- Install apps on your phone and computers to reduce blue light. For example, I am a fan of F.Lux for Macs and Twilight for Android.
- Use 'after-sunset lighting' in the house as much as possible: candles and low-blue-light-emitting bulbs for the bedroom, dual bulbs for the living area, dimmers.
- If you must watch TV, have the screen as far away from you as possible, rather than using your laptop or phone in bed right next to your face.
- Try investing in some 'blue-light-blocking' glasses if you must be on a screen at night or watching a movie at home in the evening.

The Effects of Caffeine on Sleep

Caffeine is a neurostimulant, meaning it speeds up the brain. Caffeine is also the most widely used addictive substance in the world, with up to 90 per cent of US adults consuming it daily. It increases the brain's pleasure and reward chemical dopamine, as do alcohol and other addictive substances that make you want more of them. Most importantly, when it comes to affecting sleep, caffeine binds in the brain to something called adenosine, which is a brain chemical that makes us feel sleepy and slows down brain and nervous system activity. Adenosine is like the brain's 'braking' system. Caffeine blocks adenosine and keeps us feeling more awake by removing those brakes.

How much caffeine affects you and your sleep is highly variable from person to person, due to huge genetic variation in how quickly and effectively your body can break down (metabolize) and get rid of (excrete) caffeine. There are specific enzymes in the liver that break down caffeine. The one called CYP 1A2 handles most of the caffeine breakdown and how well this enzyme works and how much of it you have is again highly individual. That is why some people can get away with drinking coffee in the late afternoon and still sleep well (although many people who claim this in fact still do have some sleep dysfunction from caffeine when you really dig into their sleep patterns!) while others are more sensitive and must avoid any source of caffeine after 11 a.m. to avoid sleep effects. Some people cannot tolerate *any* caffeine at all without it disrupting their biological clock and sleep to some degree. Exhausted-warrior types are the sort most likely to have ultra-sensitivity to caffeine, but any type can also have this since there is *so* much individual variation, far more than just the four resilience types.

It's not just coffee that contains caffeine, but also other substances such as: tea, chocolate, energy drinks and matcha. Tea has an amino acid called L-theanine which can slightly buffer caffeine's 'jacked-up' effect but it doesn't speed up how well or fast you can get rid of the caffeine so it's not a licence to consume more caffeine, especially if you are particularly sensitive. It is very common for most patients to deny or be unaware of their caffeine sensitivity level and the only way to find out is, unfortunately, to wean yourself down from and then off caffeine completely for a minimum of two weeks (ideally four weeks) and monitor what happens to your sleep quality. Notice I say sleep *quality* here, not sleep time or trouble falling asleep, because that's not typically how caffeine affects sleep the most. Caffeine tends to affect our deep sleep, called Non-REM sleep, which happens a while after you fall asleep initially. NREM sleep is actually the most important phase of sleep for replenishing your brain-chemical peptides: such as your 'happy hormone' serotonin and the feel-good/reward one called dopamine, and is also needed to repair your cells and get rid of bad or old cells (e.g. prevent pre-cancer cells from multiplying, etc.).

This delay effect on the sleep cycle from caffeine is the reason why if you want to take a power nap during the day of only twenty minutes but want to avoid dipping into deeper sleep states (which can leave you feeling groggy and worse instead of more refreshed after the nap), drinking a small cup of coffee will allow many people, especially if overtired, to fall asleep for that initial twenty minutes before the caffeine kicks in and jolts you awake before the deep sleep starts. I do not, however, recommend using caffeine for the naps on a regular basis because of its potential to affect sleep that night as well, even if used in the early afternoon.

I have had multiple patients referred to see me by their family doctors for insomnia and related issues such as chronic fatigue with poor sleep, who are still consuming some daily caffeine. They have usually been told by a well-meaning doctor that a bit of morning coffee/tea/caffeine wouldn't make any difference to sleep as long as they avoided caffeine 'in the afternoon and evening'. These patients are normally sent to see me to have an assessment for something such as medical cannabis to substitute for the often high doses of sleeping pills they are taking. They are often deemed to have 'treatment-resistant insomnia'. In other cases, due to patient preference, they want to avoid long-term daily use of sleeping pills and want to explore other alternatives. In most cases, I explain that a caffeine holiday is still necessary even if they are only having a bit in the morning, to rule out the high likelihood of caffeine playing a role. Once we overcome their initial reluctance, we discover in nearly all cases that after a four-week break their sleep has noticeably improved. To test the role of caffeine once they are feeling better, usually a few months later, we then introduce a single serving of caffeine of their choice first thing in the morning and see what happens. At least eight times out of ten, there is a negative response in the sleep pattern.

If you are an exhausted warrior or wound-up warrior, I strongly recommend doing at least a four-week caffeine holiday to help the nervous system return to a calm, restored baseline, which is essential for resilience.

If you slip up, don't beat yourself up, just start again the next day and avoid having more caffeine after the first cup. You can also take 200mg of L-theanine in a supplement form to help calm the nervous system back down a bit and add a few capsules of silymarin, a botanical extract from milk thistle, which may help support the liver enzymes, including the ones involved in breaking down caffeine. That is my 'caffeine emergency rehab' protocol. If you drink more than one cup of coffee or other caffeinated drinks each day, minimize caffeine withdrawal symptoms (which will still likely happen to a lesser extent and can include irritability, foggy headedness and sleepiness, but should go away within five to seven days of stopping caffeine) by cutting down by a quarter-cup of coffee every two days, until you're consuming no coffee, or by half a cup of tea a day. Swap it out with herbal teas, especially one with an adaptogen quality, which helps us handle stress, such as holy-basil tea (also called tulsi). To help with boosting energy and mental clarity that you may feel you are missing from caffeine, you can add some adaptogen herbs or mushrooms, such as a supplement with a combination of cordyceps, lion's mane, reishi, herbals like ashwagandha, liquorice root and eleutherococcus and/or American ginseng. Try to avoid panax, or Korean ginseng, during the day as I find this tends to be too stimulating for most people, and stimulation is what you are trying to avoid by cutting out caffeine for the time being.

The Effects of Alcohol on Sleep

The second most common substance which affects sleep after caffeine is alcohol. Alcohol's effects in the brain, we now know from advanced brain-imaging studies, are much more complex than we realized even ten years ago. Alcohol is the most socially acceptable intoxicant and most people enjoy having a drink or two because it has a rewarding effect on multiple brain chemicals like dopamine (the reward chemical), GABA (what makes us feel warm and relaxed) and our brain opioid system (pleasure and decreased feelings of pain of all sorts). That's why it's such an enticing way to 'unwind' in the evenings after a long, stressful day. However, after the initial burst of feel-good chemicals, alcohol unfortunately has many downsides in the brain and for our resilience. It can increase anxiety, especially if you are a wound-up warrior, increase chronic fatigue and depress immune function (exhausted warriors), worsen low moods and motivation (moody warriors) and impair cognition (i.e. thinking clearly) and problem-solving as well as mental clarity (scattered warriors). But most importantly, like caffeine, alcohol messes with sleep.

Even that one glass of wine or two to unwind after dinner has an effect on sleep that night, and despite it making you feel relaxed, it can actually rob you of sleep in two sneaky ways: it decreases the REM dreaming phase sleep so that you 'crash' into the next stage of sleep and it also decreases your total sleep time. REM sleep is important for helping us consolidate and process the events of the day and is thought to be important in mental and emotional health (and hence resilience). Total sleep time is just as it sounds: the total amount of sleep you get at night, a big factor for feeling rested in the morning.

For these reasons, if your resilience is low, I recommend taking at least a four-week holiday away from all alcohol.

Ideally you would continue this alcohol-free holiday for a period of eight weeks. If that feels like a very long time stuck in mocktail land, start with four weeks and reassess how you feel at the end of this period and whether you would like to see what happens by going another four weeks. I find by approaching this process with curiosity and a 'let's see how it goes' attitude, people are more likely to stick with it longer in the end than if they aim to be super-rigid from day one. Also telling your friends and family that you will be taking a break from booze as part of your resilience programme is a very important step so that they can support your process. Of course, since this book isn't medical treatment or advice, if you are worried you may have alcohol dependence, you should always seek professional help.

I realize this may sound like the 'no-fun' programme, but it's not for ever, just a short experiment. Of course, the reality is that most of our social customs revolve around these two substances – meeting up for a coffee or a drink with friends, or attending a dinner party involves the mutual sharing of them and enjoying that social aspect of life is also a key to resilience. However, once you have taken your holiday from caffeine and alcohol, you will have an idea of how much each of these substances affects you, your mood, energy levels and sleep and be able to decide how much to incorporate them back into your life and how often.

'SLEEPY FOODS'

While foods can't work like a sleeping pill, there are certain foods that are high in an amino acid called tryptophan which may help induce a sense of calm relaxation and be helpful choices for the evening meal and, if needed, a snack after dinner:

- Poultry: chicken, turkey, duck
- Complex carbohydrates: wholegrain bread, brown rice, potatoes, sweet potatoes (eat with poultry for dinner)
- Avocados (mix with greens, nuts and salmon for Dinner Salad)
- Tree nuts: almonds, cashews, walnuts, pecans, macadamia nuts
- Yoghurt and honey with banana
- Wholegrain crackers with nut butter
- Full-fat organic cow or goat's milk (warm frothed milk with honey *or* as cold drink with wholegrain crackers or nuts as a snack) *or* oat milk for a vegan option

Your Sleep Environment: Light and Sensory Reduction

In addition to getting rid of all sources of blue light in the bedroom by unplugging or covering with black tape any indicator lights or flashing lights from chargers, you want to make your bedroom as calming and soothing for your brain as possible. These are some ways to enhance your sleep environment without spending a ton:

- Get blackout blinds – any light pollution can alter sleep cycles so your room should be as pitch black as possible. You can get cheap blackout curtain liners for under fifty pounds for even big windows, to put under your fashionable ones, or pull-down blinds for as little as fifteen to twenty pounds to fit most windows. For travel or as a quicker or more temporary solution (also great for children's bedrooms!) you can get blackout curtains that fix directly onto the window with suction cups for around twenty pounds.

- As much as possible, keep your bedroom 'sacred' for sleep and sex – no work in the bedroom ideally. However, if you have young kids or the bedroom is the only place for a home-office desk, limit the hours of work so that you stop before dinner – and absolutely *no* laptops or phones in bed at night for you and/or bedpartners.
- Get a white-noise machine for the bedroom – voice-activated speakers work well, with ocean sounds on low volume, and there are free apps available on your phone that work even when your screen is dark and your phone is set to airplane mode, for an option that is both portable for travel and free.
- Eliminate clutter in the bedroom. If you are like me and are messy, hide the mess and clutter in storage areas, closets or however you can so it's not in your line of sight while in bed. These subconscious environmental factors can trigger mental anxiety or worries before sleep.
- Consider a good eye mask for total blackout, or one made from all natural silk fibres (which I prefer, along with my silk pillowcase – my most indulgent bedroom item but totally worthwhile!).
- Get good ear plugs. Flare Audio Sleep Pro are great as my investment/high-end choice, and for cheap and cheerful (and nearly as good), look for foam 38 db highest-noise-rating ones which cost around ten pounds for a hundred and last for ages if you are prone to losing them.

Supplements and Herbal Sleep Aids

The place to start when it comes to resetting sleep is by removing things first that impede good sleep, from the caffeine and alcohol to blue light, and then adding relaxation (your breathing practice for this week: see page 189). However, for those who suffer from more stubborn sleep issues, like many of my patients, 'taking something' for sleep is often needed.

I often start with very gentle herbs and supplements used in synergistic (meaning they help each other work better) combination. Supplements are the icing on the cake and it's really important to do all the other things mentioned above first. However, in addition to changing your sleeping habits, some supplements can be a huge helper. One of the issues with over-the-counter sleep supplements is that most of them just aren't effective. This is due to the dose being wrong, the formula being cut with cheap fillers, the wrong part of the plant or subspecies being used, or because they are single herb supplements only – which tend not to work as well as specific sleep-boosting supplement combos. This is one of the tenets of botanical medicine, that herbs work together quite well, especially certain ones, and generally you would choose a main herb and then add 'helper herbs' to that. Luckily for most of us who are not expert herbalists, there are many examples of these products that are pre-made. My favourite ones tend to be professional-grade supplements that offer higher doses of each herb, but for ones you can buy without a prescription, these are some of the herbs to look for, in some combination together (at least three ideally):

- *Passionflower*
- *Skullcap*
- *Lemon balm* (Avoid high doses used daily if you have low thyroid as it may lower it further)
- *Valerian* (Note: in approximately 10 per cent of people, it can have the opposite effect and make you feel awake or even 'wired', so observe your reaction over the first few days/doses to ensure this is not you. In the majority of people where it is useful, it can take weeks to start working its magic, e.g. take it for four to six weeks, because it acts on our GABA receptors and the effects seem to build up gradually in some people more than others.)
- *Hop flowers*

In addition to these botanicals, the following supplements can also be added alongside the herbals for a better effect:

- *L-theanine* – an amino acid which helps relaxation
- *Milk protein hydrolysate* – this is from cow's milk and has been shown to aid sleep in animal models
- *5-HTP* – an amino acid needed to make serotonin. It may help improve sleep based on some animal models, but the research is thin. However, some people do find it helps, especially when combined with other sleep ingredients.
- *Magnesium glycinate or threonine* – these are well-absorbable forms of magnesium, that can help with muscle tension and are considered to support mitochondrial (cell-energy) function. Many patients report it also helps with anxiety and feeling 'wound up' (hello, wound-up warriors!). When we sleep, the cell membranes in the brain open up a bit to allow more magnesium to flow in, which is why I put magnesium in the 'sleep-support' supplement category and it should be taken before bed. Normally a 400–600mg dose is used, but in some people under medical supervision occasionally more may be used, but not before checking things like kidney function.

Melatonin

Melatonin can be taken as a supplement in addition to what the brain makes naturally. It is sold as a supplement in many countries such as Canada and the US, but currently requires a doctor's prescription in the UK. I sometimes prescribe it alongside other sleep supplements and herbals and will often use a slow-release form where available, to avoid wake-ups if the issue is more staying asleep or fragmented sleep. Melatonin taken on its own is not always as effective for most people, unless it's being used to reset after flying across time zones for jetlag.

Over-the-counter Drugs

Over-the-counter drugs such as some antihistamines are often used as a sleep aid, but they should not be used for this purpose generally as they can disrupt healthy sleep architecture and may have memory-impairment effects if used frequently as a long-term sleep aid. If you have restless legs syndrome (where you feel the urge to move your legs to get comfortable) antihistamines can make it worse.

Prescription Sleeping Pills

If you have disruptive sleep issues, your doctor may suggest prescription sleeping drugs, normally only for a short time. I try to avoid using these medications for long-term regular use due to the high risk of side effects and possible longer-term effects on the brain. However, in some cases they may be needed and some drugs are safer than others and more appropriate for different types of sleep issues and other related issues like chronic fatigue and pain. For example, low-dose trazodone in cases of severe chronic fatigue syndrome can help reset sleep, often combined with sleep herbals and supplements, and then gradually decreased once sleep has been on track for normally a period of three months. Low-dose naltrexone used in conditions such as fibromyalgia may also help improve sleep.

CBD and Medical Cannabis for Sleep

Over the counter hemp CBD: CBD can help with lowering stress and anxiety levels, two sleep saboteurs. Taking a ton of CBD on its own (known as 'CBD isolate') right before bed may actually make some people feel wakeful, although not everyone. It increases the brain's wakefulness centres in some animal studies. That is why it's best used throughout the day, or in the afternoons and early evenings to help lower stress and possibly even cortisol stress-hormone levels to help your brain and body wind down properly in the hours before actual sleep time begins. You can look for a 'full-spectrum' product too, which tends to work better than isolated CBD due to what is known as the entourage effect or herbal synergy. Other cannabinoids like CBN and terpenes like myrcene may also help. You can also use CBD products combined with other herbal sleep helpers and with melatonin which tends to make it work better for sleep and evening stress.

Medical cannabis containing THC is something I also prescribe for my patients with more severe or treatment-resistant insomnia. It can be extremely effective and is usually very well tolerated with minimal if any side effects when done under expert doctor guidance. With my patients, generally I usually start with what I would consider a 'micro-dose' of 1–2 mg of THC. An oil or tincture form by mouth is usually used if the issue is fragmented sleep and waking up. Especially for those who have chronic pain that keeps them up, since it helps with that too. Besides THC, the products also contain a smaller amount of CBD to help buffer any potential THC side effects as well as other minor cannabinoids and terpenes, again like that calming terpene, myrcene. Strains for night-time are often labelled as 'indicas' although technically that is now not accurate as all the plant genetics have been interwoven over the years. In Canada and in some parts of the US, this type of cannabis oil with THC can also be purchased without a prescription at legal cannabis shops.

If the issue is just getting to sleep, I often will use a medical cannabis flower product that is inhaled with a vaporizer. Again, looking for so-called 'indica' strains in a flower form which are then ground and put into a herbal cannabis vaporizer and used before bedtime, often alongside a calming relaxation meditation or mind–body practice. This way of using it doesn't last as long as taking an oil by mouth, so it is only generally helpful for people who have trouble getting to sleep but then sleep deeply once they finally do drift off. It can also work well for those who may be especially sensitive to THC and be more susceptible to morning grogginess with an oil, although this side effect usually does improve as you get used to it and with the right dose.

SLEEP APNEA

If you snore, or your bedpartner says you do or that you make gasping noises sometimes when you sleep, and have daytime tiredness, you should get checked out by your doctor for a condition called sleep apnea. Sleep apnea is a sleep disorder more common if you are over your ideal weight but can happen even if you are slim. It is also more common as we get older. Sleeping with a portable breathing machine for sleep apnea if you do have it can completely transform your sleep resilience. Sleep apnea is often not asked about at the doctor's office unless you bring it up, so if you are a snorer it's a good idea to get checked.

Sleep Reset Protocol for All Resilience Types

- All screens off at least two hours before bedtime – for the next four weeks.
- Change blue LED bulbs in bedroom and living room to lower blue-light options: incandescent bulbs or blue-blocking light bulbs
- Eat dinner by 7.30 p.m. latest. The ideal time may be even earlier, around 6.30 if that is possible for your work and/or family schedule. This is because late big meals can cause the cortisol stress hormone to shoot up at night and impair deep sleep cycles. If you get hungry later on, have a snack from the list of High-tryptophan foods – see page 94.
- Cut out caffeine and alcohol. Wean down first if you are having more than one serving per day. Swap the alcohol for CBD mocktails and GABA-enhancing alcohol-free spirit to get the effect without the drama.
- Do your resilience breathing before sleep (see the mind–body chapter for how to do it, p. 189).

- Lights out by 11 p.m. *latest*. Sleep before midnight is better than sleep after midnight for most people, due to our clock genes.
- Avoid using your snooze button. If you must use an alarm, put the alarm on the opposite side of the room, so you have to get up to turn it off, and set your alarm for as late as possible instead of earlier with some 'snooze' alerts, since the snooze time is not helpful for contributing to restorative sleep. I like the Lumie alarm or one similar as it wakes you up gently if you tend to need a bit of a graduated wake-up.

Although following all of the tips above is the best and fastest way to improve sleep, there are specific things that may be most important to focus on for your type.

- Wound-up warriors generally have the most trouble getting to sleep. For these types, I advise starting your evening wind-down routine a bit earlier than you are used to, shutting off screens early and doing a short relaxation mind–body practice (see the mind–body chapter for best practices for your type, page 181). Along with calming mind–body practices, calming supplements like L-theanine and CBD to help decrease stress hormones may also help with getting to sleep.
- Moody warriors can have trouble with waking up very early and not being able to get back to sleep or trouble getting up in the morning at a normal waking-up time. For moody types, avoiding alcohol in the evening and, as a sleep aid, getting bright light or a lightbox in the morning as soon as you wake up may be helpful.
- Scattered warriors more often than other types may have a hard time going to sleep consistently before midnight, as in setting an early bedtime. If you are a nighthawk and are able to sleep in and generally sleep well, it may not be something you need to change. However, if it is negatively impacting your life and you want to be able to get to sleep earlier on a regular basis, having a regular bedtime routine and slowly shifting that bedtime by fifteen minutes every five to seven days may help your brain

adapt to an earlier bedtime slowly and gently, so that you start to feel tired earlier. Sometimes, under medical guidance, a small dose of melatonin in this transition period can be helpful, or taking a sleep supplement an hour before you want to be going to sleep.

- Exhausted warriors may be most at risk for having light, unrefreshed and fragmented sleep, with issues waking up in the night multiple times. Cut out all caffeine completely and avoid alcohol after dinnertime, as both can cause fragmented sleep in different phases of the sleep cycle even if they seem to help you get to sleep (alcohol) or have no impact on getting to sleep (caffeine). Using a blackout eye mask, white noise and earplugs may also help you to sleep more deeply. Sometimes sleep supplements can also make a big difference for light sleepers.

CHAPTER FOUR

THE RESILIENCE DIET

'Let food be thy medicine and medicine be thy food'
Hippocrates

Dan came to see me for low mood and fatigue. He was frustrated because he had tried medications, eating healthily and exercising more, which seemed to help at least a bit at first, but over time these interventions gradually lost their effect and he felt like he was 'back to square one again'. He knew he had a good life: a stable job, a healthy relationship and two young children. He didn't have severe, crushing 'can't get out of bed' depression or full-blown chronic fatigue syndrome. However, his low mood and energy had a big effect on his happiness. He managed to 'seem happy', as he put it, when with friends, so not many people knew he was suffering. We started him on a lower-carbohydrate/higher-fat 'keto-lite' whole foods diet, removed gluten and other possible food-intolerance agents, and started a gut-healing protocol with foods after discovering his microbiome was less than optimal on stool testing and testing for leaky gut. These are two common functional medicine investigations I utilize because we know now that gut health, food, mood and energy are all related. We also started a few natural supplements to help with gut health and energy. Six months later, his mood and energy scores were improved, he said he felt like his brain had 'woken up' and he had more of his mental faculties at his fingertips again. He also had less trouble getting up in the morning and more motivation, which allowed him to start a short morning-exercise home regimen, which he had tried before but was never able to stick to. He also had more energy. He gave up alcohol for an initial eight-week period and now stuck to having only a very occasional drink since he just felt 'clearer' and had fewer mood ups and downs even though he was never a binge drinker previously and only drank in moderation. When he came off his diet on a two-week holiday, he felt his mood and energy issues creeping back towards the end of the vacation. So he restarted the diet as soon as he returned, with the mood and wellbeing benefits thankfully also returning. Nine months after revamping his diet, we redid his microbiome testing and discovered that his leaky gut as well as his bad bug to good bug ratio had dramatically improved, and many of the gut 'red-flag' markers associated with low mood and fatigue were returning to normal.

Although depression and chronic fatigue syndrome are not 'nutritional illnesses' with a single root cause, changing the diet and working on improving the microbiome health can make a big difference. Often, in addition to changing the diet, medications and/or other integrative approaches are needed too. Diet alone is often not enough to tackle low mood, poor energy and lowered resilience especially if the issues are severe. However, gut health and gut microbes have a huge influence on our mood, energy levels, immune system and cognition (or thinking). By altering our diet and, in many cases, adding specific supplements, we can shift how healthy that gut balance is and have a positive impact on each of these areas. These changes tend to 'hold' as long as you stick to the diet most of the time, but tend to start to slip if bad eating habits return.

If leaky gut and leaky brain are suspected, there are more specific food and supplement interventions based on more advanced functional medicine tests as well as symptoms which can be explored with a doctor trained in integrative or functional medicine. This is the approach I take with my patients. If the blood–brain barrier becomes leaky, as happens with leaky gut, food proteins and other substances we ingest that should be trapped in the gut get absorbed and cross into our bloodstream in the body and then may travel one step further into the brain, leading to an inflammation cascade. This low-grade inflammation may contribute to a whole host of resilience issues for every type: anxiety and toxic stress in wound-up warriors, autoimmune issues and chronic fatigue in exhausted warriors, depression in moody warriors, and brain fog, poor focus and memory in scattered warriors.

The fact that the gut is so crucial to both physical and mental wellbeing and resilience is not a new concept. Ayurveda, the ancient Indian system of medicine, considered gut health to be the core focus of all health and treatment and that when the Agni fire (which we may consider in modern terms to mean digestive ability and gut wall health, i.e. no leaky gut) was low, disease resulted. And what affects one person's gut one way can have a different effect on someone else's. That is because we all have a unique mix of genetic factors and slightly different gut bacteria. As was the case in Ayurveda, which was focused on preventing illness before it started, or in the early stages using things like food approaches, I see food as medicine as the perfect, accessible resilience tool to use before we get sick, as part of preventative medicine. So even if you are currently feeling quite resilient, now is the perfect time to investigate your diet and what small tweaks you can make that may make a big difference to your gut and brain health in the long run.

You would think given all of the evidence on how nutrition affects our brain and body function, that doctors spend a lot of their training learning about nutrition and gut health. However, sadly this is still not the case – although it is changing slowly. It is shocking to many, but in most medical doctor training programmes, a few hours of nutrition is all we get taught in almost a decade of training. It was basically considered quackery a decade ago to suggest that gut bacteria could play a role in mental health. I did my nutritional medicine training separately from my medical degree as part of my integrative medicine training and research. Even before medical school, and in fact one of the reasons I was excited to become a doctor was so that I could teach my patients how to improve their health and wellbeing using foods. Nutritional medicine and natural supplements with proven evidence behind them were a personal passion. They were tools I used myself and with my friends and family members to help them overcome health issues and also to help with energy, mood, weight management and general wellbeing. I used what I learned to help me through the sleep-deprived, stressful, clinical-doctor trainee years in order to avoid downing ten coffees a day like many of my peers. I then started using what I knew to help my patients, who often had never discussed nutrition before with a medical doctor beyond the vague 'just eat healthily' advice that did little to guide them.

What Does the Science Say?

It's not just what we eat either but what time we eat, how we eat it (i.e. taking time to not rush through meals in a state of distraction) and how much space we leave between our last food before bed and our first meal in the morning that can contribute to how our diet affects resilience. There are some universal core principles to stick with that will benefit every resilience type. Then, based on your type, there are some specific things you may want to consider.

There are so many diet fads out there that it's hard to keep track of them all. They almost all promise an almost instant or 'overnight overhaul' that is simultaneously easy to stick to long term. This is a really sexy, tempting idea and I totally understand the appeal of the instant body transformation. However, the reality is that most dietary changes take time to take effect, involve habit and behaviour change and can be really tricky in a fast-paced life where it's not always possible to cook from scratch or avoid eating out or on the go. Making dietary changes that are sustainable in the long term is, in my experience, all about making one or two small changes at a time in most cases. Crash diets don't work: they are impossible to stick to in the long term and often do more damage than they fix due to creating the feeling of deprivation which leads to bingeing and an 'Oh, screw it!' mentality after feeling constrained for too long – and often hungry too – on an impossible regimen. Crash diets also take the joy out of eating and we know the joy of sharing food and socializing is important for overall resilience.

It is very difficult to make major multiple changes at once, and not everyone will need the exact same diet. Based on the combination of your resilience type and individual needs, you may need to stick to some of the resilience-diet principles more than others to reap the most benefit. For example, not everyone needs to be on a strict gluten-free diet, but many people who don't have coeliac disease still may suffer from non-coeliac gluten sensitivity (NCGS, page 110). Hence, for many people, cutting out gluten as a single diet change can help with issues ranging from brain fog and fatigue to food cravings. You may also choose to make a different change, cutting out, or drastically reducing, sources of added sugar from your diet (e.g. sweetened drinks, candy and sweets) and get your pudding fix by making some healthier options like date- or fruit-sweetened energy balls or unsweetened dark chocolate. Or, if that seems too extreme, you may choose to add something in, such as three servings per week of high-omega-3 small fish (such as herring, sardines or mackerel) or one more serving per day of green vegetables. You may also decide to swap one thing directly for something else, for example, caffeinated coffee for Swiss Water decaf to decrease your caffeine intake. It's up to you and your lifestyle.

It also takes some personal experiments to see what makes a difference for you. If, for example, you experiment with cutting out all gluten for six months and don't notice any positive effects, then you might well decide that is not something you want to continue long term. If, however, you reduce added sugar and find you have better energy levels week after week, it will motivate you to continue swapping healthier whole foods for refined sugary ones. The more positive changes you make – and stick to – over time in alignment with the core principles of the resilience diet, the better you will likely feel. Even though diet change is hard, it really does matter what we do (and don't) put into our bodies and brains for fuel.

So as you embark on potentially making some dietary shifts for resilience, be kind to yourself, start gently and be patient so that you can incorporate these changes in a way that feels as natural as possible rather than a punishment or exercise in self-control or 'willpower', which just doesn't work in the long run. It's not about making all of the changes at once but, instead, choosing one (or a few if you feel up for it!) and trying it out for a month or two first, seeing how it makes you feel. Some of the changes, such as cutting out gluten grains if you are sensitive to them, may take six months or even longer for maximum benefits, so patience is key.

This process also means introducing your body and taste buds to new flavours, textures, foods and ways of eating that may seem completely alien to you right now. But the process can become enjoyable as you discover new foods and pleasures which are tasty as well as healthier and your tastebuds will get 'retrained' and adapt over time.

Normally people find that as they make changes to what they eat, gradually things that they considered a 'treat' previously, such as sugary drinks, processed foods or desserts are no longer appetizing and are replaced with healthier 'treats'. For example, desserts with an unsweetened dark chocolate base, or organic berries with a small amount of fresh organic cream, kale chips roasted in the oven replacing packaged potato crisps, etc.

No matter how big or small the changes you decide to make, the number-one rule is 'no guilt'. If you start a change and you slip up, no beating yourself up or convincing yourself that you are a bad person or feeling guilty. If you tend to have a cycle around guilt and dieting from past experience, choosing a self-compassion meditation for your mind–body practice is highly recommended (see the mind–body chapter for details, page 181), especially if you are a moody warrior.

Eating for Resilience Core Basics

These are the core principles of what I call the 'resilience diet'. In reality, this is more of a way of approaching food and helping your microbiome out rather than a quick-fix 'fad diet'. These are core ways to start using foods as medicine for all types:

- Ensure that the majority of the food you eat is low on the GI score – aka the glycaemic index. The GI is a measure of the sugar load of a certain food. The lower the score, the better the food is for you and your blood-sugar balance. Choose most of your foods for each meal with a GI score of 40 or lower. Eating lower-GI foods helps keep blood-sugar levels balanced, which is critical to brain health as well as preventing issues like Type 2 diabetes and metabolic syndrome and can also help keep weight in a healthy range without calorie counting or dieting.

- Eat vegetables at most meals and make them as colourful as possible. Even at breakfast, incorporating things like eggs (or tempeh or tofu) with spinach or chard with organic butter or olive oil drizzled on top is a nice way to get some more veg in before lunch. This is not the typical 'healthy' breakfast we have grown up to imagine, which has been based on ads for 'healthy granola' for the past forty-plus years. In India, a typical breakfast consists of dahl, which is curried lentils with fresh herbs. But for those of us who don't have time to cook in the mornings, a green smoothie or green juice alongside organic sourdough with flax, organic butter and often some fruit and goat's yoghurt is a quicker way to sneak in some veg before noon.

- Think of meat as a 'side dish'. If you do eat meat (I personally do), still try to make veggies plus legumes and a smaller amount of healthy wholegrains cover most of the plate. The type of meat you choose is important too. Wherever possible, choose meat that is organic, grass-fed (for beef), free-range (chicken) and organic outdoor bred (pork). Trying to avoid 'factory-farmed' meats is important in terms of both carbon footprint and the health effects.

- Eat more high-fibre foods. Especially soluble fibre, but both soluble and insoluble fibre types aid digestion and can help general gut health and provide food for the healthy gut bacteria. Soluble fibre is found in flax, apples, avocados, legumes (beans) and pears just to name a few sources. Swap 'white' carbs with wholegrain 'brown' carbs, e.g. wholegrain pasta, rice and bread instead of white, to increase your fibre intake with the same meals as you already eat.

- Be aware of your gluten intake, especially in processed 'white' carbs. Not everyone is sensitive to gluten, however it is one of the food proteins most likely to affect the gut lining and may contribute to a leaky gut over time. Gluten-containing foods are those which contain wheat or wheat flour. Even if you do not have coeliac disease, there are many other immune-related 'intolerance' reactions to gluten that may have a similar effect on the gut, making it leakier and contributing to many vague symptoms. This cluster now has a medical term – non-coeliac gluten sensitivity. I have found that exhausted warriors are the most likely type to feel best on a completely gluten-free diet, but any of the other types that also have brain fog or fatigue as an ongoing issue may want to consider cutting it out completely.

- Eat Lots of Healthy Fats, especially the 'big three':
    - Medium Chain Triglycerides (MCTS), which have special properties including helping with fat-burning and blood-sugar regulation. Virgin cold-pressed coconut oil is a good source of MCTS.
    - Omega-3 fatty acids. Omega-3 fatty acids are one of the most important brain-resilience foods. They are brain protective as a group and the three main types – eicosapentaenoic acid (EPA), docosahexaenoic acid (DHA) and more recently docosapentaenoic acid (DPA) – each have their own unique brain effects and also work together. EPA and DHA are found in fatty fish, such as herring, mackerel, anchovy and salmon. Try to stick to smaller fish, since heavy metal mercury levels tend to be high in king mackerel, white albacore tuna, and swordfish. Choosing wild salmon over farmed is preferable since another bioaccumulation called PCBs may be present in significant levels in farmed salmon, due to contamination of the feed for the farmed salmon with PCBs. You need two to three servings per week to get the brain benefits ideally, although for many people this is quite hard to do, especially if you hate the taste of fish or hate cooking it, so supplementing in a pill form may also help (see the next chapter, page 157).

- MUFAs (Monounsaturated fatty acids). These are richest in oils such as olive oil, cold-pressed canola (rapeseed oil) and avocado oil. These MUFAs have potent anti-inflammatory effects in both the brain and body which make them superstars for all resilience types. Although MUFA oils are also higher in omega-6, they are still very healthy oils to include alongside your omega-3s as they are not 'inflammatory' like refined vegetable oils, for example.

- Choose low-'AGE' foods (or reduce high-AGE foods). AGE stands for 'advanced glycosylated end products', but the acronym is also appropriate because foods high in these AGEs also age your cells, create free-radical damage and inflammation and therefore are 'anti-resilience foods', no matter what your type is. High-AGE foods are highly refined foods such as processed meats, cold cuts and frozen pizzas, 'junk' breakfast items like baked goods and pastries, as well as snack foods such as cookies and fast food like fried meats, fried chicken burgers, French fries or fish and chips. A diet high in these foods makes it much harder for your cells, brain and body to cope with stress of all varieties and leaves you more vulnerable to resilience busters for each type. Really watch out for your intake of these foods if you tend to eat out a lot or eat on the go, because home-cooked foods tend by their nature to be lower in AGEs than grab-and-go meals.

- Choose foods high in glutathione building blocks. Glutathione is the master antioxidant in the brain and body and helps fight free-radical damage as well as make more energy inside each brain and body cell. Pre-formed glutathione is not in any one food (though you can take it as a supplement: see page 240), but the building blocks to help the body make more of it exist in specific foods. Making sure you eat these regularly will help your body keep up its supply. Each group of foods helps us make glutathione, by supplying a key building block as follows:
  - Sulphur-rich foods: sulphur is needed to make glutathione and it comes from beef, fish and chicken (highest sources)

and also vegetable sources such as cruciferous veggies (cauliflower, broccoli, Brussels sprouts), alliums (garlic, onions, shallots) and leafy greens such as mustard greens, kale and chard.

- Selenium (which is a mineral needed to make glutathione work properly in the body): found in foods such as beef, chicken, fish, Brazil nuts, cottage cheese and brown rice.
- Whey protein, which is high in cysteine, an amino acid needed to make glutathione. This comes from cows and is a powder that can be used as a base for smoothies or added to kefir or yoghurt.

- Eat a rainbow and avoid 'monochrome' meals as much as possible. Fruits and vegetables of different colours are rich in plant 'super-compounds' like anthocyanins and polyphenols that help buffer oxidative stress in our cells and enhance our resilience, immune system and protect our DNA and telomeres from shortening. Each vegetable and fruit has its own mix of these super-compounds, so the more variety and colours of fruit and veg you eat, the more of them you will get.
- Include fermented foods to support a healthy microbiome. These include foods such as kefir (which has a higher probiotic content than yoghurt), yoghurt, kimchi, sauerkraut and miso, just to name a few. For most people without specific intolerances, these foods can fuel a healthy gut flora balance.
- Reduce toxins, chemicals and synthetic ingredients as much as you can. Avoid any food-label ingredient you cannot pronounce or that is a name of a synthetic chemical such as the E-number dyes and food additives, as well as artificial low-calorie sweeteners, binders and preservatives. This includes reducing the amount of residue from pesticides and herbicides by trying to choose unsprayed or organic options whenever possible.

Is Organic Really Better?

The answer is yes, but not in the ways you might think. Many studies have shown there are not significant differences in vitamin and mineral content between conventionally grown produce and organic. However, organic produce has been shown to have higher phenolic compounds, which are powerful plant antioxidants called phenolic phytonutrients. These may help reduce free-radical damage in our cells too, just like they do for the plant. It's also about what is *not* in organic produce. Even though pesticide residues can still be in organic produce, they appear to be much lower. Many pesticides may also affect our mitochondria (the energy factories) which is why it's important to reduce exposure to help keep our cells as resilient as possible, especially if you are an exhausted-warrior type. A new study has shown that three common pesticides used on fruit and veggies do in fact disrupt hormone balance, especially oestrogen balance, so this is another reason to choose organic or 'unsprayed' whenever you can, especially for women's health issues, regardless of your resilience type.[1]

What About Dairy?

When I first started prescribing nutritional medicine, aka food as medicine, for my patients a decade ago using an integrative medicine framework, it was very common to advise patients to reduce cow's-milk dairy products because they were thought to be 'pro-inflammatory' in many natural-medicine circles. But the science has changed recently, and so has my advice.

It has been discovered that any type of animal-derived milk (ideally you would want to stick to organic milk from grass-fed cows in healthier pastures) seems to be potentially anti-inflammatory, according to some research studies,[2] or at least neutral. This is even the case if you already suffer with a low-grade chronic inflammation: dairy intake did not have any adverse effects such as increasing the inflammation in another study.[3] Dairy of all types, as a food group, may also be brain protective and help increase brain levels of glutathione, the most important antioxidant for resilience.

Fermented dairy, such as kefir, which is sort of like thinner drinkable yoghurt, yoghurts, and quark, as well as fermented cheeses such as Camembert, are better as a resilience food than plain milk. There are specific compounds, such as two called oleamide and dehydroergosterol, in fermented dairy products that researchers have identified as responsible for reducing the risk of Alzheimer's dementia by reducing microglia (the special immune brain cells) inflammatory responses and neurotoxicity, two ways dementia attacks the brain. Other recent studies concluded that fermented dairy may reduce the risk of cognitive decline and dementia. A number of studies have found that low-fat dairy as a general group appears to be brain protective as we age.[4] However, to muddy the waters, a recent Swedish study suggested that high intake of cow's milk (i.e. non-fermented dairy) was associated with an increased all-cause risk of mortality (death from all causes) via a specific cell-signalling pathway, which conflicts with the other studies saying that cow's milk is likely anti-inflammatory or at least neutral.[5] The other long-held advice given to patients by doctors since the early 1980s was to choose low-fat or 'skimmed' milk and low-fat dairy, yoghurt, cheeses, etc. over the full-fat versions and to reduce their intake of butter, another high-fat dairy product, because of supposed increased risk of heart disease. However, the research since has shown that full-fat dairy does not elevate the risk of heart disease, and in fact may reduce the risk. So even if you have a strong family history of heart disease, avoiding high-fat dairy is not necessary.

Some people who find they may be sensitive to fresh (unfermented) cow's milk find they tolerate a specific type of cow's milk better. This is called 'A2 milk', which has a different protein. There is some possible weak evidence that some people may be less sensitive to this A2 protein as opposed to the more common A1 version. Cows in the south of France and in the British Channel Islands, for example, naturally produce more A2-type milk. In practice, I have found some patients over the years tolerate this A2 milk better, but some just do better without any cow's milk at all.

It is possible to have an allergy to one of the milk proteins and that is definitely a reason to avoid it. However, in patients who suffer with eczema (very dry skin) dairy seems to be a trigger even if they don't have a milk protein allergy. Conventional dairy may also contain residues of antibiotics if the cows had been sick, or in some countries (this is not allowed in the UK or EU currently) the cows are also given hormones to help them make more milk and these can also end up in the milk too. Then there are those pesky environmental pollutants, POPs and other chemical residues to think about, which is a valid concern after scientific evidence has demonstrated that these do enter milk.

In summary, the research around dairy and its health benefits is often confusing and even contradictory. The bottom line so far is that moderate intake of dairy is fine for most people, but fermented dairy is best and organic is important to decrease the exposure to bioaccumulant chemicals. If you get gut symptoms like bloating and gas after eating dairy products, it is likely you are lactose intolerant. You can try choosing lactose-free milk or fermented dairy and cheeses and taking lactose enzymes with dairy products if you want to keep dairy a part of your life. I also have some patients who do much better on a dairy-free and 'casein-free' (a milk protein) diet, especially if they suffer with ADHD or similar 'scattered warrior' issues.

With dairy, as with most dietary approaches, what works for one person may not work for the next. Become your own 'food detective' by trying one or two small changes at a time and see how you feel over the next eight to twelve weeks. If you want to see if dairy does affect you, you could try cutting out all dairy completely or a more gentle change like swapping cow's dairy to goat's dairy (which may have slightly more easily digestible proteins) and sticking to mostly fermented products like yoghurt over milk.

Top Resilience Foods to add to your diet	Foods to reduce
Lower-sugar fruits, especially berries and non-tropical fruits like apples and pears	Added sugar/refined sugar/sugar in its many forms, including fructose, high-fructose corn syrup, glucose, etc. (check food labels)
Nuts and legumes	
Cruciferous and sulphur-rich vegetables	
Green leafy vegetables	Processed foods with preservatives, anything you cannot pronounce, colourings, artificial flavourings, carrageenan
Root veggies high in soluble fibre	
Herbs and spices	
Small fatty fish, wild not farmed	Breads and foods made with white or 'wheat flour,' 'wheat' or white bread (sourdough bread is the best 'wheat' choice as it may help break down the gluten protein and may make it less likely to cause a food intolerance)
Gluten-free wholegrains like quinoa, amaranth, millet and buckwheat, wild rice and brown rice	
Grass-fed cows, bison, venison, lamb and organic free-range chicken in 'side-dish' amounts	Processed meats from cold cuts, hot dogs, salami, deli meats, sausages
Healthy oils: cold-pressed virgin coconut oil and olive oils, organic butter and ghee	Baked goods
	Fast foods
	Deep-fried foods
Fermented foods including vegan sources (tempeh, miso, sauerkraut and kimchee, fermented organic dairy like kefir and yoghourt, dairy-free yoghurts)	Bottled fruit juices, sodas and drinks with sugar
	Refined carbohydrates: pastries, white pasta, cookies, snack crackers, crisps, white bread/wheat-flour breads

Food intolerance

There are some people who have a very clear-cut typical allergy to certain foods, meaning when they eat them they become covered in hives or get facial swelling, wheezy and, in very severe cases, can have trouble breathing. This is only one type of food reaction, which is caused by IgE allergic antibodies in the immune system. Until recently, it was believed that food intolerances were 'just digestion issues' and doctors routinely told patients that they were 'not immune-system related'. However, more evidence has emerged to suggest food intolerances may involve the immune system in many different ways and contribute to a host of gut and non-gut symptoms (e.g. mood-related symptoms, anxiety) in some sensitive individuals. Other types of food issues and intolerances may be related to issues processing a chemical called histamine, or by contributing to leaky gut in the case of some proteins from wheat like gluten.

So how do you know if you may have food intolerances? The best way is still to do what is called an elimination diet. That is when you cut out a food you suspect you may be reacting to for at least two to four weeks (I recommend at least six weeks for most things since it may take more time to see a change) and then slowly reintroduce that food back into the diet, eaten twice a day. If you are testing more than one food that you cut out, only reintroduce and test one food at a time before moving on to the next one every three days, to avoid cross-reactions. Unfortunately, even current functional medicine tests for food intolerances do not replace a good elimination diet when it comes to finding out what foods may not be a good match for you. If you suspect or have been diagnosed with MCAS (mast cell activation syndrome) or another histamine-related issue, a more extensive approach is usually needed, such as a low-histamine diet and in some cases medications and/or natural supplements to stabilize the mast cells and reduce the histamine intolerance to foods over time. I have had many patients over the years who had undiagnosed symptoms of MCAS and responded well to a low-histamine diet. This can be explored with a health practitioner skilled in this area of medicine.

Going 'Keto'

I'm going to start by saying I *love* bread. Not that horrible white sliced bread or anything close to processed. But nothing makes me happier than starting the day with a slice of good sourdough with some organic nut butter and flax seeds. A good loaf of bakery sourdough is my top comfort food.

Which makes the emerging body of research showing the benefits of a lower-carb plus high-fat diet as possibly one of the best ways to eat to slow brain ageing and reduce the risk of dementia slightly depressing for me and, well, most other people. I've adopted a keto diet for short stints in the past before childbearing years, out of a combination of convenience (my husband follows this dietary strategy so it made cooking and meal planning easier!) but have never made it a fixture as my default way of eating. I've never needed to, because I've been lucky not to suffer with a mood disorder, cognition issue, chronic fatigue syndrome or autoimmune condition like many of the patients I treat in my practice. These are all conditions where a keto diet may be worth trying.

Ketogenic diets can improve chronic fatigue syndrome/ME symptoms in many patients, although big studies to prove this connection are still lacking. One of the reasons why they are still lacking is that the diet is also a bit of a hard sell to doctors, who are normally already sceptical of 'dietary' interventions as medicine and also generally lack an up-to-date understanding of chronic fatigue syndrome/ME. Then you have to convince patients living with chronic fatigue to cut out many of their favourite foods because they are too carby. When you live with chronic fatigue, your life has already become very small, with the inability to do many things that bring joy, like exercise, going out and socializing and having meaningful work and passion projects, because you are so incredibly fatigued. Food is often the only comfort or thing to look forward to in their day that is left open to these patients. And because it's a food approach, no drug company is getting excited about sponsoring and paying for the dietary research because it's not patentable. I digress, but you get the picture.

So why take this seemingly extreme step if you already have a healthy diet? If you suffer with a chronic condition related to brain and nervous-system function, have a high familial risk of early dementia or if you are a moody warrior and you suffer with depression or frequent low moods, these conditions are associated with abnormal insulin regulation in the brain and may benefit from a keto style of diet, based on preliminary research and case reports. Specifically, areas such as the hippocampus and the amygdala, the brain areas for learning, memory and stress regulation appear affected by diet. A low-carb, high-healthy-fat diet may help normalize or improve the function of these brain areas, hence alleviating the brain fog and cognitive dysfunction as well as improving tolerance to stress in people with issues like treatment-resistant depression, for example. Ketogenic diets also appear to help restore normal microglial (the brain immune cells we learned about in Part One) function in rats with depression, something that is thought to work in humans too although the research is only preliminary. Certainly working with patients who have overlapping diagnoses of depression, immune dysfunction and fatigue, I have found that ketogenic-style or modified types of this diet called 'keto lite' plus taking ketone supplements (see next chapter) can make a huge difference to all these symptoms for many people.

These low-carb, high-fat diets are not new in medicine, despite the fact that most doctors know very little about them. They have been used for a hundred years as part of a treatment for epilepsy and, more recently, many other conditions that would fall under the neuropsychiatric category, such as depression, bipolar and chronic fatigue syndrome/ME as well. They have even been trialled alongside chemotherapy in some cancers to possibly sensitize the tumour to chemotherapy and decrease the toxicity and side effects from the cancer drugs.

The word ketogenic comes from the fuel-source shift that your brain goes through when you stop eating lots of carbs, which normally provide sugar in the form of glucose to the brain and body. Instead of glucose, when that is in short supply the brain and body start to use ketone bodies instead. These are made in the liver when it converts fat stores or fat from the foods you just ate into an alternate energy source – aka the ketone bodies. That is why generally a keto diet is high in fats, since this is where the energy comes from. Having protein intake too high can also put additional stress on the kidneys especially if you already have kidney issues. And last but not least, not enough fat can leave you feeling hungry, on edge and stressed out, which is again not what you want. So having a higher fat intake helps you feel full longer and avoids carb cravings. That's how a keto diet differs from some of the other 'fad' high-protein diets that restrict both carbs *and* fat, which can leave you feeling chronically hungry and unsatisfied.

After you start using these ketone bodies for fuel, it appears they are brain protective, as long as you stay in what is called 'nutritional ketosis' or light ketosis. Unless you have Type 1 diabetes, it appears so far to be pretty safe for most people, generally speaking (of course always check with your doctor first since a book cannot offer individual medical advice).

The keto diet may, over time, decrease food cravings and appetite. This type of diet also appears to be mitochondrial protective, meaning it keeps your cell-energy powerhouses functioning at their best. This is extra-important if you suffer from a condition which affects the mitochondria, like the chronic-fatigue/ME spectrum of illnesses as well as post-cancer-treatment fatigue even years after remission. One pathway ketones work on is related to turning off something called the 'inflammasome' in the brain, a set of proteins responsible for activating inflammation. The keto diet may also work by improving resistance to stress and free-radical damage in the brain as well as helping with 'brain housekeeping', namely getting rid of old cells. It can also help with brain ageing. People at higher risk for developing Alzheimer's – that is, older adults starting to have slight memory complaints – found going on a keto diet improved not only their memory and cognitive scores but their actual brain chemical markers for dementia in the spinal fluid.[6]

In this way, the ketogenic low-carb, high-fat diet is quite similar to another treatment I use a lot: medical cannabis. They both can improve seemingly unrelated conditions and both have been received with scepticism by many doctors unfamiliar with the research. However, they are both becoming more widely accepted as part of a more holistic yet still very much evidence-based approach to treating these complex chronic conditions where a magic drug cure does not exist.

It may not be necessary to go 'full keto' to reap many of the benefits, and how far you need to go with them also seems to be quite individual. I like to think of the most practical version of what I tend to recommend to people who want to try this style of eating as 'keto-lite'. If you are an exhausted warrior, a keto-lite diet may help improve your energy levels and make it possible to do things like exercise again and expand your 'energy envelope' or use more energy points each day without feeling exhausted again. If you are a scattered warrior, this way of eating can help with focus and reduce food cravings over time.

The Keto Diet for Women

When I first started researching the potential benefits versus the downsides of a ketogenic or even 'keto-lite' diet, the first thing that sprang to mind as an integrative medicine practitioner who treats lots of women was how would this diet impact our cyclical hormone cycles, especially since many early studies on keto diets were done on men? What about for women trying to get pregnant, for example? How does this diet affect healthy women who want to do something more 'preventative' as opposed to women who already had existing hormone imbalances like polycystic ovarian syndrome, metabolic syndrome/prediabetes or obesity? And what about the effects of the diet for perimenopasual and postmenopausal women? The research in many of these areas, sadly, is still in its early days and largely lacking in the published literature. However, some data does exist. In a study with overweight women with PCOS, a keto diet improved hormone balance, insulin (blood-sugar balance) and healthy cholesterol levels after twelve weeks.[7] This is in line with what I have seen clinically over the years with PCOS patients adopting this diet before trying to get pregnant, with resulting improvements in how they felt and possibly improved fertility.[8] Another study in women with hyperinsulinemia who were overweight showed that a ketogenic diet improved all aspects of blood-sugar control, triglyceride levels (a measure of unhealthy fat in the blood) and reduced BMI (i.e. weight loss) and that in women with pre-diabetes who are overweight the keto diet could be recommended as part of medical treatment.[9]

However, the keto way of eating, like any dietary approach, may not suit everyone. Some women may find it worsens their mood or anxiety levels when they go 'low carb' and that the stress this causes isn't worth the potential brain-ageing benefits. One small study in healthy women showed that after four weeks on a keto diet compared to the control diet (normal western diet), women reported feeling more fatigued with daily tasks. In contrast, I have found that many women (and men!) who suffer with chronic fatigue/ME and similar low-energy conditions, such as fibromyalgia, get an increase in their energy levels after going on a keto or 'keto-lite' diet. This may be due to people suffering with chronic fatigue/ME-spectrum illnesses actually having biological differences in the way their cells use energy, and that using ketones for fuel instead of carbs may help their cells use energy more effectively.

It is also possible for diets too low in carbs to cause period problems or disrupt normal healthy menstrual cycles in some women, based on anecdotal evidence. This is something I have seen too over the years, especially in women who are not overweight and usually with the high-protein, low-carb and low-fat 'fad' diets rather than keto, but it's something to look out for.

This is, again, why diet is such an individual thing. Even within resilience types, there is lots of variation in how people respond to this style of diet. This is an occasion where doing your own 'N of one' trial is beneficial. This means you are 'patient number one', as in only one person in the little study you are conducting for yourself, and keeping track of what happens each week so you can assess after one and three months if you've noticed any positive changes as well as negative reactions. I like this approach because part of becoming more resilient is becoming your own 'resilience scientist'.

Intermittent-fasting Windows

For resilience and brain benefits, you can also employ an eating strategy known as intermittent fasting. This is often talked about alongside a keto diet, but it can be done alone with any healthy diet too. It can take many forms, but the type I am talking about and recommend to people is having a longer than average period of not eating in every twenty-four-hour cycle. This can range from twelve to sixteen hours of 'fasting' and then the rest of the day, i.e. eight to twelve hours, is your 'eating window'. The other ways to do this are to fast for one whole day each week, or even more often, e.g. a thirty-six-hour fasting window. The problem with the latter approach is that most people find it very impractical to fit into a normal lifestyle, especially when trying to do normal things like share a meal with your family or friends and also have enough energy to get through the work week and then enjoy your weekends. The research is also pointing to these bigger, whole-day fasting windows as being potentially beneficial for men but potentially detrimental to women, due to gender differences in how this fasting window affects insulin sensitivity (improving it in men versus making it worse in women in one study)[10], but the research is still in its early days.

How to Do a Full Keto Diet

Generally, a full keto diet involves getting around 70 per cent of your total daily calories from fats, 10 per cent from carbohydrates, and 20 per cent from protein. If you get too much protein combined with not enough carbs and not enough fat, you can end up feeling constantly hungry and unsatisfied, which can lead to food bingeing. So getting enough fat is important to the success of this dietary approach. This hunger feeling is one of the main reasons why lower-fat, low-carb, high-protein diets for weight loss were not sustainable in the long run and most people ended up stopping and regaining much or even most of their weight lost in so-called 'get slim quick' commercial weight-loss approaches that used this approach.

How Many Carbs Can I have?

If you are shooting for a full-on ketosis effect, e.g. the strict 'medical version' of the keto diet, the answer is not many – 20 grams or less a day.

However, this is usually not necessary or practical for most people, unless it's a medically supervised diet for controlling epilepsy or to try to help reverse or stall the brain changes seen in Alzheimer's dementia.

The Keto-Lite Resilience Medicine Version

I have found when I work with people on their diet to enhance health and wellbeing, it's really important to keep it realistic and not rob some-one of the joy of food. It's also what is sustainable for you in the long run, because if you feel deprived, you will not stick with this style of eating for very long and are more likely to have a 'f— it' carb-gobbled binge day eventually. This is why I like to call my version 'keto lite'.

The 'keto lite' is done by keeping carbs below 100 grams per day and having those carbs mainly coming from non-starchy vege-tables and a small serving of lower-sugar fruits plus one or two small servings per day of a wholegrain (e.g. quinoa or brown rice) or len-tils. Making sure those carbs are healthy, whole-food carbs and not sugar or refined carbs is super-important. That is because the fibre in healthy carbs like wholegrains, veggies and fruits decreases the amount of insulin that gets released, which has an effect on blood sugar and ketosis too (less insulin released = more ketosis).

One way to get those ketone bodies with a few more carbs seems to be adding in more medium chain triglycerides into the diet as a common keto-diet 'hack' or shortcut. These take the form of MCT oil or virgin cold-pressed coconut oil. MCT oil doesn't have the coconutty taste and has no smell, so you can put it into foods, drinks, coffee, sal-ad dressings, etc. without knowing it's there taste-wise. Some people do a combination of the two. Having 15ml or 15g of MCT oil three or four times a day, which equals a daily amount of 45–60g (60g is used in some studies), tends to work well for this enhancement effect. That means you can still have quinoa porridge in the morning or a serving of your favourite wholegrain with dinner and eat more root veggies while still getting the positive keto-lite effects. Even though MCT oil is high in fat and calories, it does not generally cause weight gain. In fact, it seems to help control blood sugar and may actually have a beneficial effect on maintaining a healthy weight.

MCT oil drinks have become popular with keto-diet enthusiasts as a morning breakfast substitute. The drink combines black coffee or tea, organic butter and MCT or coconut oil all mixed in a blender to create a super-rich zero-carb, high-energy drink with a caffeine hit. This is certainly a way to maintain ketosis until lunchtime and also tolerate a bit of caffeine without adverse effects. Generally, this drink for 'breakfast' strategy is best suited to moody and scattered warriors. If you are a wound-up or exhausted warrior, skipping the caffeine is the best idea or substituting Swiss Water decaf. Even decaf coffee does not agree well with most exhausted warriors, despite them often drinking multiple cups to get through their day, as it usually causes energy crashes later in the day and fragmented sleep. If this sounds like you, substitute it with a coffee-free version made with turmeric instead and add herbal adaptogens such as a medicinal mushroom blend, liquorice root and Siberian ginseng in the morning to help with energy levels instead (see details in the next chapter on supplements for each type). Many exhausted warriors may find they feel more fatigued if they don't eat food in the morning. Wound-up warriors may find that not eating till noon makes them feel more anxious. So skipping breakfast is not for everyone. It is something you may have to experiment with to find what works best for you.

What to Eat

So you may be thinking, *OK, I'm sold, but what the heck can I actually eat now and how do I learn to cook all these things without spending an hour or more in the kitchen every day? The* good news is there are delicious things to eat, including things that we may have thought we needed to avoid for health reasons, like organic cream, cheeses, eggs and cooking with healthy oils like cold-pressed olive oil, coconut oil and organic butter. There are also a plethora of relatively quick recipes that require less than fifteen minutes and only a few ingredients to get started. (I recommend getting a few good keto cookbooks and also a paleo cookbook which is 'grains free' and will be lower in carbs too just by virtue of not having recipes which rely on grains primarily.) There are also no-cook things like cheese or nut-butter dips and veggies and smoothies for quick meals (something I make use of a lot!). We have grown up thinking of 'cutting carbs' as a weight-loss 'diet' and many associate it with feeling deprived, hungry or missing out on the joy of foods, but when you really up the fat content, you may feel more satisfied than you did on a high-carb, low-fat diet once your body adjusts over a few weeks' time.

The healthiest way to do the keto-lite diet is by making sure you still eat mostly whole foods and minimize processed and fried foods and max out the veggies in a rainbow of colours. This ensures you are getting all the key micronutrients you need and the fibre to avoid constipation and keep the gut healthy and happy, since when you dramatically reduce grains you remove a main source of fibre and minerals from the diet. Even though they do contain carbs, for most people I do not recommend strict 'carb counting' or restricting most vegetables and low-sugar fruits (all berries, avocado, citrus fruits, grapefruit being the lowest, kiwis, peaches, cantaloupe and water-melon, in 1 cup servings) due to their multiple resilience benefits. Root vegetables (potatoes, yams, sweet potatoes, winter squash, parsnips) and higher-sugar fruits can still be eaten but in smaller amounts since they have a lot more carbs. This is generally known as a more 'Mediterranean keto diet', where vegetables, fish and small amounts of legumes are encouraged (green beans and black soy-beans are the lowest carb and therefore good ones to go for more regularly or for a bigger serving). So again, this version is really 'keto-lite' as it is much higher in carbs than a very strict, traditional keto diet, which means if you pee on those home ketone strips, they may not show you are making many ketones. If you are keeping the carbs under 100g a day and the fat content high as well as using the keto hack of adding in more MCT oil and/or ketone supplements, that should still give you many of the benefits. It will also feel a lot less restrictive for normal life, including eating out with friends and not becoming an obsessive carb counter.

How a Resilience Diet Actually Works to Change the Gut and Brain

If you want to know some of the science behind how the resilience-diet way of eating works, it can be broken down into what I like to think of as seven key areas. Even if you succeed in shifting just one of these areas with a small change in how you eat, it can make a massive difference to how you feel.

- Balancing blood sugar and reducing insulin resistance. This is important because impaired fasting blood sugar from eating a high-sugar-load diet not only leads to Type 2 diabetes and cardiovascular (i.e. heart) disease, but also is now linked with premature brain ageing, dementia, depression and chronic fatigue syndrome.
- Increasing cell energy and supporting detoxification pathways. Inside each of our cells, as we learned in Part One, we have kidney-bean-shaped things called mitochondria. These little beans are the energy factors in the brain and body. It turns out that how well they work is determined by a mix of genes plus environment – including what we eat and put into our bodies. There are many genetic differences, called SNPs, or single nucleotide polymorphisms, which affect how sensitive our little energy factories are to resilience busters. That is why some people may be able to get away with a much poorer diet than others, depending on how sensitive they are and their unique SNP combination. This sensitivity can also change over time. Especially if you are an exhausted warrior, you tend to need extra support in this area. One way to support our mitochondria is by making sure there is lots of glutathione floating around. Glutathione is the most powerful antioxidant in the body and helps make our mitochondria function better. It also decreases damage from free radicals and supports liver detoxification of everything we ingest, from pesticide residue to food ingredients to drugs (prescription and recreational ones

including alcohol), and also aids in heavy-metal detoxification. Healthy glutathione levels also protect against premature ageing by protecting our telomeres, the little hats on the end of our DNA that determines our lifespan essentially, by controlling how fast our cells age. You can take it as a supplement (see the supplements chapter, page 141) but also get the building blocks from your diet.

- Regulate and reduce inflammation. Neuro or brain inflammation, microglial (brain immune cells) regulation and global chronic inflammation all contribute to mental and physical health symptoms which zap resilience for all types. Reducing the pathways of chronic inflammation and supporting microglial function through an anti-inflammatory diet is key to health and also to getting chronic inflammation-related symptoms under control. Many forms of depression are now thought to be related to brain inflammation (moody warriors!) as are chronic fatigue spectrum conditions, which likely involve dysfunctional inflammatory control pathways.
- Optimizing the microbiome and gut health. We now know that the types of bugs in our gut and the ratios of each type do not only affect our digestive system as we previously believed. Psychobiotics, as we learned in Part One, is the term for how our gut microbes have a direct impact on our brain and mental health too. Unhealthy gut bacteria contribute to leaky gut, which can lead to inflammation and wreak havoc in our body and, potentially, in our brain too, by allowing food and chemicals to cross into the bloodstream and over the blood–brain barrier where they trigger an inflammatory response and immune reaction. This can cause issues for every resilience type and symptoms such as burnout, anxiety, fatigue, low moods, problems with focus and memory and many seemingly 'unconnected' symptoms.
- Provide quality building blocks to make brain peptides. We need to get our building blocks to make things like our happy hormone, serotonin, and all of our other important brain

neuropeptides, or brain chemicals, from our diet. This means when the diet quality is lacking in a key element (say, omega-3 fatty acids), it has a negative impact on how well we can build healthy brain chemical levels that support mental wellbeing, mood, energy and resilience.

- Reduce toxin exposure. Herbicides, pesticides, persistent organic pollutants, microplastics and many other things that we have not yet evolved to deal with well all enter the system through our digestive system via food. These chemicals disrupt hormone systems, the gut lining and gut microbes, even the blood–brain barrier and affect our brain-chemical balance as well as creating an extra stress burden on our cells. Hence, trying to choose organic or 'unsprayed' produce where possible and drink filtered water is key.

- Protect our telomeres. Telomeres, part of our DNA or genetic code, can be thought of as little caps on the end of our DNA, you'll remember. They control how fast our cells age when they get shorter over time. Certain foods are thought to be telomere 'protective' while others may contribute to shortening these caps and degrading them, leading to premature cell ageing and increased risk of major chronic illnesses and low resilience states.

PEARL BOX: REDUCING HORMONE DISRUPTORS FROM FOODS

There are many hormone- and endocrine-system-disrupting chemicals that we can get exposed to from our diet as well as other sources like plastics, coated non-stick cooking pots and pans, cosmetics, cleaning products and home furnishings. These chemicals imitate our natural hormones and bind to receptors in our body and even brain and have been linked to hormonal imbalances, infertility and neurological symptoms. For the dietary offenders, many of them are so persistent now in our food chain and soil that they are impossible to avoid altogether. However, we can reduce them by trying to do the following as much as possible:

- Buy organic or unsprayed whenever possible, especially for the 'dirty dozen'.*
- Invest in a water filter jug and, if you can afford it, a reverse osmosis filter that is installed on your tap.
- Try to avoid lots of canned foods, stick to dried when possible or if you do buy canned beans, for example, look for brands that say 'BPA free', although some of these may still contain other similar chemicals.
- Swap 'non-stick' pots and pans for stainless steel or cast iron, pottery or glass.
- Avoid storing food, especially hot foods, in plastic containers and avoid reheating things in plastic. Go for glass instead where you can.
- Try to reduce and avoid where possible foods with artificial dyes, flavourings and preservatives by choosing whole-food alternatives where you can. Some food dyes, such as tartrazine, are still common in many foods and cosmetics in the UK although it has now been banned in other countries, such as Norway due to its wide-reaching potential health effects on everything from neurological function and fertility to microbiome health, based on animal models.

Additional Eating Tips for Your Type

In addition to the core resilience-diet principles, there are some additional dietary things you can consider to support your specific resilience type.

WOUND-UP WARRIORS

Because calming a 'wound-up' nervous system is your challenge, you want to specifically support a calm balance via foods and drinks. The calming brain chemical called GABA may be in short supply in

---

* https://www.ewg.org/foodnews/dirty-dozen.php

wound-up warriors, so adding foods rich in the GABA building blocks may help. GABA is the neurotransmitter in the brain needed for feeling calm, being resilient to stress and being able to shut off constant anxious or worried thinking.

Increase/eat more of these:
- Fatty fish (i.e wild salmon)
- Legumes
- Organic eggs from chickens and ducks
- Organic chicken
- Turkey
- Oats/oatmeal
- Yoghurt and kefir (organic, full fat and unsweetened, e.g. plain). To make the taste a bit nicer without adding sugar, you can add a dash of vanilla extract and/or liquid stevia.
- Millet
- Fermented soy products (i.e. tempeh, miso)
- Brown rice, quinoa
- Tree nuts and seeds
- Water and herbal teas (mild dehydration causes an anxiety reaction in the body)
- Steamed (or raw) deep leafy greens with olive oil as a regular side dish at meals
- Deep leafy greens, salad greens
- Extra virgin olive oil for salads
- Cold-pressed coconut oil (for cooking)
- *Specific foods high in taurine, which is an amino acid needed to make GABA:*
  - Beef, lamb, dark chicken meat
  - Eggs
  - Dairy products
  - Seaweed, krill
  - Brewer's yeast (used for baking)

- *Specific foods high in B6, which is the calming B vitamin, great for wound-up warriors:*
  - Chickpeas
  - Beef and organ meats
  - Potatoes
  - Bananas
  - Winter squash
  - Nuts
  - Non-citrus fruits
- L-theanine, another calming amino acid found in green tea, from naturally decaffeinated green tea to get the L-theanine without the caffeine hit.

Cut out caffeine completely: coffee (even decaf) dark chocolate, black (herbal tea is fine), energy drinks and supplements. Wound-up warriors are also more prone to having problems getting to sleep than other types and caffeine eveh earlier in the day if you are a slow metabolizer of caffeine can affect this without you realizing it. Even a small amount of caffeine can contribute to anxiety and a more sensitive stress-hormone response.

EXHAUSTED WARRIORS

Getting maximum energy out of your food and supporting mitochondria function is the main goal. Again, a diet high in refined, processed foods with chemical additives and preservatives may lead to worsening fatigue in many exhausted warriors, who tend to be extra-sensitive to these things. I have also found this resilience type does not generally do well on the 'raw-food' diet promoted by many wellness gurus as a cure for all chronic fatigue. This type of diet tends to be harder to digest if your digestion is already a bit pressurized. In classical Indian medicine, they call this 'low Agni fire' in the gut. I find exhausted warriors tend to do best on a cooked-foods diet of whole healthy foods, also known in Ayurvedic medicine as 'warming foods'.

I have also had many exhausted types come to see me for chronic fatigue who were on a strict vegan diet. My clinical experience has been that instead of helping the issue, it can make some people feel worse. After a sensitive discussion around their comfort level with introducing a small amount of animal protein back into the diet, we usually decide on at least a small amount of chicken and fish, from local organic and sustainable sources whenever possible. This is a somewhat controversial statement in the current climate where vegan diets are promoted as the healthiest way to eat for everyone and also as being best for the environment. However, the reality is much more nuanced. The high concentration of plant proteins in the vegan diet can cause intolerances for many people, especially exhausted warriors I find, and in the presence of a leaky gut and possibly leaky blood–brain barrier. This is where food proteins get to places where they shouldn't be and cause the immune system to react negatively. What I do love about the vegan diet, however, is how creative you can get with making veggies taste amazing, so vegan cookbooks are still a great addition to your repertoire (I love them for great ideas!) to help come up with new ways to get lots of micronutrient-rich veg into your diet, which helps decrease cell oxidative stress and free radical damage. Having a few vegan meals each week is also a great way to cut down on your meat consumption. Of course these are also general guidelines so if you are an exhausted warrior who finds a strict vegan diet is what makes you feel amazing, then continue!

- *Be aware of:*
  - Too much raw kale and too many raw cruciferous veggies. Stick to cooked due to the possibility of these foods eaten raw being 'anti-thyroid' due to compounds in them called goitrogens. Foods that can contribute to low/normal thyroid function can also worsen fatigue. Avoid putting raw kale in green smoothies
  - Any food you suspect you may have a sensitivity to. (Many exhausted warriors have hidden food intolerances, including foods that are high in histamine, or release histamine, lectins in some plant foods, or oxalates. This is beyond the scope of this book but is important for some people and is something

you can investigate with a functional-medicine or integrative-medicine practitioner to see if this may apply to you.)

- *Choose more foods high in N-acetyl cysteine or NAC, a glutathione precursor needed to make energy:*
  - Cruciferous vegetables are one of the richest food sources of glutathione, especially Brussels sprouts. Others include cauliflower, broccoli (particularly the flowers, not the stem), cabbage, kale, pak choi, cress, mustard, horseradish, turnips, swede. Just make sure they are gently steamed most of the time rather than raw.
  - Garlic and shallots

- *Minimize or cut out these:*
  - Cut out caffeine: coffee (even decaf) dark chocolate, black tea (herbal tea is fine), energy drinks and supplements. Even though it's tempting if you are always feeling tired to reach for caffeine, it leads to an energy high followed by a crash. If you are currently drinking a lot of coffee, making a change first to green tea or matcha latte, which still contains caffeine but also has the calming amino acid L-theanine in it, can lead to fewer energy crashes. Then, over time, decrease the amount of this source of caffeine too and try some non-caffeine energy supplements if you need a boost (see the supplements chapter under adaptogens and suggestions for your type, page 141).
  - Avoid a totally raw diet.
  - Avoid any foods on the 'dirty dozen' list completely unless you can get them organic/unsprayed. Choose ones on the 'clean fifteen' list* instead whenever possible as a substitute in recipes if you cannot get organic. This is because pesticide and herbicide residues may again be more of an issue to this resilience type and affect energy metabolism and impair

---

* https://www.ewg.org/foodnews/clean-fifteen.php

mitochondrial function, something that now has dozens of research studies supporting it, so is no longer 'just a theory'. Organic really is safer and healthier for you, especially if you have a fatigue-related issue.[11]

- Cut out all wheat and gluten. Many exhausted warriors have an impaired gut barrier/gut lining or 'leaky gut' and tend to be sensitive to gluten, which can open the spaces in between the gut lining cells and make leaky gut worse. This leads to more food proteins getting into the bloodstream and causing immune reactions when they shouldn't. Often this shows up as a million food intolerances on a functional medicine panel and patients have been told they are 'intolerant' to everything, but it is actually due to leaky gut playing a role and when the gut is repaired, many intolerances resolve on their own. Many people with this resilience type find they just feel better cutting it out completely.

In addition to this, exhausted warriors may do very well on a 'keto-lite' diet, but have a hard time adapting to the dietary shift for the first two to four weeks. To test it out for yourself, ideally try to stick with it for six weeks and track your energy levels to give yourself a good indication of whether this level-two resilience diet works well for you and makes you feel more energized. Those with autoimmune diseases also often find the keto-lite diet reduces their pain and inflammation and improves energy levels. People suffering with these conditions are more likely to have this resilience type, I have found.

If you have even a slightly sluggish thyroid (which you can have tested by your doctor, measuring what is called T3, rT3 and T4 levels, the three thyroid-hormone levels, in the blood), which can also cause fatigue, you may want to avoid excessive amounts of a few foods:

- Excessive amounts of raw brassicas, also known as cruciferous veggies, such as raw kale, cabbage, cauliflower and broccoli. Gently steaming them first reduces chemicals that can interfere with thyroid function so you can then enjoy them since they have many health benefits.

- Soybeans. Genistein can be goitrogenic (i.e. can cause thyroid goitres and thyroid problems in people who are prone to low thyroid or already have a thyroid problem) if consumed in large amounts as a main protein source, e.g. in some vegan diets. However, fermented soy products such as tempeh have many health benefits, so still include them, just in moderation if you have low thyroid function.
- Millet. This grain in larger amounts can also be 'anti-thyroid' but in small quantities it is normally fine.

MOODY WARRIOR

For moody warriors, many find that their diet can have a huge impact on their moodiness. This is what I have found to be the best tips for your type:

- *Eat mostly foods that are low on the glycaemic index*. This is a blood-sugar balancing diet and blood-sugar rollercoasters have a negative impact on mood and mood swings.
- Consider going keto or keto-lite. Keto diets have been used in small studies to treat depression and mood disorders and the associated fatigue that can often come with these conditions, as we touched on earlier.
- *Increase foods high in folic acid*. Folic acid, or Vitamin B9, is important for positive mood balance. Many refined grains have folic acid added to them, for example pasta or breakfast cereal, but these are generally both high carb and refined, so even on the resilience level-one diet they are best minimized. That's why it's super-important to include foods naturally rich in folic acid. We need at least 400mcg a day but I recommend at least 1mg a day for moody warriors. The top foods are:
  - Organic beef liver
  - Lentils
  - Asparagus

- Avocados
- Leafy greens (e.g. spinach)
- Brussels sprouts
- Beets
- Walnuts
- Flaxseeds
- Citrus fruits (e.g. lemon, lime, grapefruit, oranges)

- *Increase foods rich in B12.* Some studies have shown an association with low B12 and folic-acid intake and an increased risk of depression, although the research is still conflicting. However, if you are a moody warrior, making sure you are getting enough B12 from foods is very safe and possibly helpful for mood as well as contributing to a healthy brain and nervous-system function overall, since insufficient levels can lead to fatigue and anaemia.
  - Sardines, trout and salmon
  - Beef
  - Fortified nutritional yeast (this is a vegan-friendly source and can be added to many foods, marinades and salad dressings)
  - Organic milk and dairy products
  - Fortified 'mylks' (these plant-based mylks do not naturally contain B12 so must have it added – check the label!)
  - Vegan diets are low in B12, so generally supplements are recommended if you are strictly vegan.

- *Increase foods high in tryptophan.* A diet rich in tryptophan in some studies has led to improved mood in people suffering with both depression and anxiety and is easy to achieve by just eating more of the following foods:
  - Wild game meat, e.g. venison
  - Cottage cheese: goat's, sheep's or cow's
  - White, kidney and soybeans
  - Avocado
  - Organic pork, duck, turkey and chicken meat

- Pumpkin seeds
- Wheat germ (only if you are not gluten intolerant – otherwise stick to the other ones here!)

SCATTERED WARRIOR

Especially for scattered warriors, although this can also happen with moody warriors too, avoiding addictive cycles of food intake can be a challenge. Scattered warriors may be more prone to addictive behaviours, due to how the brain's reward circuits are wired. That includes foods too, not just substances or shopping binges. Addictive foods have a similar effect on the brain to other addictive substances, drugs and behaviours like gambling and binge spending. Bingeing on 'moreish' foods can be an irresistible temptation. The cycle of food cravings and in more extreme cases, food addiction, has a brain basis. It has been proven that a high-fat plus high-sugar diet leads to more food cravings. That is why it is really important if you are following a keto or keto-lite diet to avoid 'cheats' where you mix loads of sugar with fats. This 'high-fat, high-sugar' diet takes a healthy keto diet and turns it into a standard western diet, which is pro-inflammatory and anti-resilience. The combination of especially animal fats plus sugar is a recipe for inflammation. So if you are having trouble sticking to a keto-lite diet after trying it, it is much healthier to change back to a healthy whole-foods diet with carbs from healthy sources and keep the sugar low to avoid the high-sugar plus high-fat trap.

Many scattered warriors also find that intermittent fasting windows are helpful, regardless of whether they follow a keto-lite diet or not, in terms of improving focus and concentration. More than other types, scattered types, I find, are more likely to do well with skipping breakfast to lengthen the fasting period, or eating their first meal at 10.30 or 11 a.m. instead of immediately after waking. Or even trying a 'bulletproof' high-fat coffee as breakfast instead of foods and then eating the first meal around noon.

Scattered warriors should also increase their omega-3 fatty-acid-rich foods, especially from small coldwater fish or krill sources. Less bioavailable non-fish sources of omega-3s include hemp hearts, flax, chia and walnuts.

There are so many ways to use foods to help us become more resilient, starting with our gut health. Don't feel you have to go crazy and completely overhaul your diet tomorrow, especially if it feels overwhelming. You can start with one simple change like decreasing your caffeine intake, swapping white pasta for brown, or eating dinner a bit earlier to give you a bigger overnight 'fasting' window. Even just knowing that what we eat (and don't eat) can have a positive effect on our gut and brain health is a great start. When you are ready to make a food change, you now know where to start to reap the resilience rewards for years to come.

CHAPTER FIVE

RESILIENCE SUPPLEMENTS

Kristen arrived for her first appointment with me with an enormous plastic bag filled with different vitamins and supplements. She'd bought them online and from the high street, and admitted she was totally confused as to whether any of them were 'doing anything' to help the burnout she was experiencing as a corporate lawyer working constant late nights and weekends. She tended to take them a bit sporadically when her stress levels worsened, but never really noticed a difference. She also found she tended to get different advice on what supplements to take every time she went to a health shop and had ended up buying dozens of pills and potions over the years that only added to the confusion. Kristen, it turned out, was an exhausted warrior, so needed extra support in the energy department. We started by tweaking her diet, introducing a simple guided relaxation practice based on yoga nidra to listen to lying down each day, and then tackled her supplement regimen to help her get a few quick wins.

When we went through her huge bag of supplements, I discovered that although some of them were potentially useful, many had fillers, used the wrong part of the plant or wrong variety (herbals) or were in a suboptimal or poorly absorbable form of the active ingredient. Some were just totally unnecessary or at such teeny-tiny doses that they were unlikely to make much impact, if any. We slimmed everything down and started with some core basics for her type, including some energy-support supplements, sleep support and a daytime adaptogen to help with energy without making her anxious or jittery. I also recommended a full-spectrum long-acting CBD product to help with stress. After one week, she noticed she was starting to sleep a bit better and feel less *exhausted at the start of the day. At three months, she no longer had afternoon energy crashes. She didn't have to resort to candy, pastries or caffeine to keep going until 5 p.m. She was amazed at the transformation. Could we have done it without the supplements? Maybe. But many stress-related issues are improved in just a matter of weeks with carefully chosen supplements and botanicals in combination with the other core resilience-medicine tools, especially because we can't always eat and behave perfectly. Supplements and botanicals, especially in combination with cannabinoids, can give us a 'stress buffer zone' in life which is exactly what most of us in hectic modern life are looking for.*

I see so many patients like Kristen who have spent a small fortune on supplements without knowing if they made any difference. It's a confusing supplement world out there, so in this chapter I am going to help cut through the confusion to help you feel confident trying the best ones for your type. Of course, if you have a specific condition, tailoring this approach even further to your needs with a trained medical professional will give even better results but there is still so much you can do on your own too, to maximize the benefits from supplements and avoid wasting money and ending up more confused than when you started.

Supplements and botanicals are not a magic overnight quick fix for everything, but they can often give a quick win for very little or no side effects. When given in the right combination, at the right dose and using the right parts of the plant and purity, they are an important resilience tool for most patients I work with, as well as a mainstay of my own and my family's daily wellbeing regimen. A common argument for why people don't need to take supplements is that if you follow a very healthy diet (e.g. the resilience diet in the last chapter) and eat organic, there is no need for anything else: you can get everything you need from your diet alone. However, to utilize natural compounds such as botanicals, minerals and other nutraceuticals therapeutically, meaning you are using them to help target an issue such as stress, anxiety or low energy, the amounts you need to get a response are normally many times that which you can get from the diet alone. Even to meet the minimal recommended intake for most micronutrients, let alone clinical doses of them, is a challenge. In fact, the majority of the population falls short of these critical values for at least some of the key micronutrients like Vitamin C, the B vitamins and magnesium using the diet alone. I follow one of the healthiest balanced diets of anyone I know, but I still take supplements and find they make a huge difference to the way I feel, especially for my stress levels as a wound-up warrior and for my sleep.

So it may be true for a very tiny minority of people that food is all they need to feel optimal, but in my experience, most people have gaps in their resilience profile. Even for those who may feel food-based approaches alone are enough to make them feel well currently, using supplements and botanicals to enhance your resilience potential to avoid or prevent future issues you might be prone to, based on your genes and your type, can help you do that.

Based on your resilience type, targeting resilience gaps with every tool we have, especially the low-risk natural ones, is key to turbo-charging resilience and also overcoming issues that may be holding you back. For example, if you are already feeling anxious (wound-up warriors) or fatigued (exhausted warriors), you probably want to go for a 'clinically effective' dose of the specific supplements and botanicals that can help support you in those areas, and these generally need to be highly concentrated in the form of a supplement since you cannot eat enough to get to these levels normally.

That being said, many chemist and grocery-store supplements are often completely ineffective due to being very low potency, low quality, extracted from the wrong part of the plant or the wrong plant species (when it comes to botanicals) or the wrong form of the mineral/compound to be effective. Often a high-street-shop supplement will have a fraction of the active ingredient that is required for a 'clinical', meaning noticeable, effect to treat a specific symptom or even just for general wellbeing. Part of the reason for this is cost (people buy cheap stuff, it's a proven fact regardless of quality) and in some cases may also be due to allowable limits of some nutraceuticals when sold directly to consumers.

That is why in my practice I tend to use some professional supplement products for practitioners which are harder to buy directly. However, many high-quality brands are now selling direct to the public and this is becoming increasingly common. The availability of high-quality supplements in shops is also increasing, but it depends on the shop as well as knowing what to look for and how to spot the good ones on an entire wall of supplements claiming to do or be the same thing.

Another issue with many high-street-store supplements is the form of the supplement or that the active nutraceutical is not in bioavailable (e.g. absorbable) form to your body. So buying supplements can be a minefield, even with all the online information available.

To make it a bit easier to wade through all of the information both online and in a shop, there are some basic supplements that everyone or most people should consider. After looking at those, I will discuss the best supplements to consider for your type.

If you have medical conditions, it is always best to work with a qualified medical professional to make sure your supplements are both safe for you and most effective. One of the things I love about botanicals and supplements, however, is that armed with the right information and access to high-quality products, they can be a powerful and empowering self-care tool. Even after reading this chapter, you will probably know more about supplements than your own doctor, since this is another topic that is not on the medical-school curriculum.

FOR EVERYONE

Below are the supplements that are beneficial to every resilience type and regardless of what resilience level you feel you are at currently. I like to call these more core 'resilience stack'. These are also ones I take personally every day.

- **High-potency Omega-3s**
Most people who eat a healthy diet still have suboptimal levels of both types of omega-3 fatty acid, eicosapentaenoic acid (EPA) and

docosahexaenoic acid (DHA), to reach that 'golden ratio' of omega-3:omega-6 fatty acids of 1:1–1:3, as we learned about in the last chapter on the resilience diet. This ratio as well as the quantity of omega-3 fatty acids, both DHA and EPA, help with reducing brain inflammation, supporting mental acuity, positive mood and attention in concentration, as well as the ability to stay calm and stress free, hence all resilience types benefit. Because of issues with possible contamination and it being practically impossible to reach very high doses of omega-3 through food sources alone (fatty fish, the food source of EPA + DHA, may have significant toxicity due to high levels of mercury, PCBs and/or dioxins, all environmental toxic compounds that can interfere with our endocrine and nervous system), I use highly filtered, pure supplement forms of these oils from either small fish or krill. The optimal general dose for small-fish sources is around 2–4g/day, or 1g/day for krill oil.

- **Magnesium**

This is another one I add to the stack for almost every patient, unless they have a contraindication such as a kidney problem, for example. Although most of us are not severely deficient, many people have symptoms of insufficient amounts of magnesium available in our body and brain. A regular blood test for magnesium will miss it, because most of our magnesium is *inside* our cells, not in the serum of the blood which standard blood tests measure. It has been shown in research studies that screening for chronic low magnesium is very difficult because this normal serum, or blood, level can still be associated with having a silent moderate or even severe deficiency of magnesium in the body.[1]

There is currently no simple, highly accurate lab test to figure out the total body magnesium status. The best we can do currently is to test the red blood cell magnesium intracellular (inside cell) levels. This is not something your family doctor will offer you, but is normally done by a functional or integrative medicine doctor with a specialized test. However, this is pricey and hard to get on your own if you don't have a functional or integrative doctor currently on your healthcare team. Many, if not most of us, have suboptimal levels, due to increased magnesium turnover and use from chronic stress and caffeine.

Magnesium is involved in over 300 crucial chemical reactions in the body and also in protecting our cell-energy powerhouses, the mitochondria. The mild forms of magnesium deficiency are usually 'silent' or asymptomatic and signs that mainstream medical doctors look for are absent or non-specific, ranging from trouble getting to sleep to fatigue and brain fog. (While these symptoms are usually from a complex cause and not eliminated by supplementing with magnesium as the only intervention, in most cases it does tend to help them and in some cases makes a huge difference.) Chronic low-grade magnesium deficits increase the free-radical damage in our cells which have been associated with many chronic illnesses including heart disease, high blood pressure, Type 2 diabetes, depression and stress-related conditions as well as dementias, just to name a few.[2]

There are many different forms of magnesium. For example, if you suffer from chronic constipation, magnesium citrate can be a good option since it helps replenish magnesium stores as well as relieving constipation as it works as a natural laxative. For brain resilience, and especially for exhausted warriors as well as scattered warriors, magnesium threonate may cross into the brain over the blood–brain barrier much more easily than other forms to possibly help with cognition and focus memory and also appears to enter the mitochondria, the cell-energy powerhouses, to help them function better.[3] Sometimes, I will use a combination of the citrate form and the threonate form – for example, in an exhausted warrior type who also suffers from constipation-dominant irritable bowel syndrome to get the dual effects. Magnesium biglycinate or glycinate is another good form I use often with my patients and it's easier to find and much cheaper than the threonate form.

- **Multivitamin (High Potency)**

One of the most common supplement questions I get asked is 'Is a multivitamin worth taking?' My answer is always the same: it depends on what's in it and how much. If you are a woman who is of child-bearing age and thinking of getting pregnant, already are pregnant or breastfeeding, a multi-formulated pregnancy and breastfeeding supplement with extra folic acid and the right amount of iron, making sure it doesn't have too much Vitamin A, is worthwhile. There are also men's health variants with slightly different trace elements that may be important for prostate health in men.

- **Vitamin D**

Vitamin D is one of the most underrated supplements and one of the most essential single nutrients to sustain health and resilience. It's actually not just a vitamin but also a hormone too, involved in regulating critical functions in our cells, brains and bodies. Vitamin D deficiency is very common. Billions of people are affected worldwide and most of them don't know it because there are no symptoms for many years. However, deficiency is linked with nearly every major chronic illness, ranging from cancer, diabetes, bone and heart disease to autoimmune diseases and neuropsychiatric illnesses (which involve the nervous and immune system, like fibromyalgia, chronic fatigue syndrome and chronic Lyme) as well as depression and mental-health conditions.

The importance of having optimal levels cannot be understated. It is an easily accessible and inexpensive key nutrient that supports so many aspects of mental, physical and immune-system health. Since Covid-19 first occurred, it has been in the spotlight more often because lower Vitamin D levels have been linked with higher death rates from Covid and risk of severe Covid-19 infection and it appears that supplementing may be protective.[4] I put all of my patients on Vitamin D, with very few exceptions. Because Vitamin D is a fat-soluble vitamin, meaning it is not well absorbed unless with a fat, you need the oil version, not the pill (unless that pill is an oil-filled capsule, which is fine). Between 1,000 and 5,000IU per day of Vitamin D3 is the general dosage range for most people, although in some cases on the medical side of things I use a higher dose. Even babies need supplements if they are breastfed, since breastmilk is pretty much the perfect food for the first months of life, except it is low in Vitamin D. With my son River, I used the infant Vitamin D oil at first and now that he is weaned, I give him a combination omega-3/Vitamin D oil supplement on a spoon each day.

PEARL BOX: THE LINK BETWEEN VITAMIN D AND MAGNESIUM

Due to increasing awareness about Vitamin D insufficiency in the majority of the population, even mainstream medical doctors not trained in nutrition are starting to recommend routine supplementation. This is great news, but may be having a negative effect on magnesium, which is needed for the body to process the Vitamin D – and as we just learned, most people are also magnesium deficient too to some degree. That is why taking both together is so important.

- **Probiotics**

Probiotics are living microorganisms, usually bacteria but sometimes beneficial yeasts, which when taken in high enough amounts on a regular basis create a health benefit in humans, via the gut which is the 'host' environment for these microorganisms. This basically means they are good bugs that you can put into a capsule and take as a supplement. If you suffer with digestion issues like irritable bowel syndrome, you may already be taking a probiotic or at least have heard about their benefits. However, in recent years, researchers have discovered that probiotics are not just for gut health. They support a healthy gut microbiome, which is the genetic material of over a trillion microbes living inside your digestive system. This collection of bugs is actually like its own organ since they communicate directly with the brain and nervous system and impact at least most of the brain's neurochemicals which control things like our mood, as well as send signals to the immune system.

In order to have optimal brain functioning (e.g. a resilient brain), you need to have the best bugs in the mix, which may not always be possible from diet alone. Probiotics may also improve mental health, lower inflammation, improve blood-sugar balance and improve our antioxidant capacity to fight free-radical damage, as well as improve other metrics of health related to resilience, according to recent studies.[5,6] Probiotics may even be able to enhance bone health (by improving bone mineral density) in post-menopausal women.[7]

The explanation for these wide-ranging benefits is likely related to the gut–brain–immune-system axis. As we learned in Part One, a healthy gut supports a healthy brain and immune system and vice versa. So for their potential wide-ranging health benefits and the fact that they are generally extremely safe and well tolerated, I consider them part of the core 'resilience stack' for most people. I recommend looking for a high-quality 'broad-spectrum' probiotic that is 'shelf stable', but still keeping it in the fridge so that it remains as active as possible once opened. Occasionally, for specific health issues, I may custom-order specific probiotic strains, or types, after doing a functional-medicine stool test to see what the community of bugs looks like and how it may be best to alter it. But in general for healthy people, a good-quality general all-rounder probiotic will do.

Blood-sugar balance and food cravings

Wound-up warriors and moody warriors tend to be prone to more carb or sugar cravings when they get out of balance, but any resilience type can have this issue. Chromium is a supplement that has research-proven evidence to help balance blood sugar and curb cravings for carbs and sugar. This is obviously part of a sugar and food craving reduction plan alongside food approaches (see the previous chapter, page 103) and mind–body stress-reduction approaches (see the mind–body chapter, page 181):

Dose: chromium picolinate, 200mcg twice a day.

All About Adaptogens

Because bad stress is a universal resilience zapper for all types, it is also worth considering adding some herbal adaptogens. Adaptogens are botanical extracts that help the brain and body adapt better to chronic stress. They do this by helping to regulate the HPA axis. In order to be an adaptogen, an herbal extract must also have low toxicity, be non-intoxicating and non-addictive. Each traditional medicine system has its own adaptogens based on the plants that grow naturally in different parts of the world. Each adaptogen is slightly different too. In botanical medicine, we call this uniqueness the plant's 'herbal signature'. That means some adaptogens may suit one person better than others. However, some are quite helpful for all types such as:

- **Full-spectrum CBD extract (Cannabidiol)**
CBD is an adaptogen as well as a cannabinoid. It appears to help regulate our stress and cortisol response in the brain, especially when in a full-spectrum form with all of the other bioactive minor cannabinoids and terpenes to make it generally more effective at lower 'wellness' doses. Stick to a high-quality full spectrum CBD oil twice a day. Also see the cannabinoid chapter for more details (page 159).

- **Eleutherococcus senticosus (Siberian ginseng)**
This is a very different botanical from panax ginseng (aka Korean ginseng), which is more likely to cause overstimulation or jitters. The active plant compounds appear to help regulate stress-hormone production and may even downregulate genes associated with an exaggerated stress response over time. It may also help improve immune response under stress. Dosages vary by product.

- **Withania somnifera (Ashwagandha/Indian ginseng)**
This is an Indian Ayruvedic botanical used to help regulate the adrenal stress hormones and activity and also is a potent antioxidant. It is not too stimulating and in fact is considered to be calming adaptogen. It is also my favourite go-to adaptogen for women's health. I have also used it for borderline low-thyroid with lots of stress: there is not much published evidence, but I've found it useful. Dosage-wise, you can take up to a few grams a day of ashwagandha root, but you can start with 600mg since everyone's dose will vary slightly and also varies based on the formulation (as with all botanicals).

Supplement Stacks for Your Resilience Type

In addition to the general stack that is beneficial for most people, specific supplements based on your type can help enhance your resilience based on your type-specific challenges, since each type is slightly different. If you are a combination of two types, you may benefit from the suggestions in both areas, starting with the suggestions for the most troublesome area for you. (For example, if fatigue is the number-one issue, focus on those supplements first for three months or so to avoid supplement overwhelm and to know what is helping with what.)

EXHAUSTED WARRIORS

If this is your resilience type, the supplements to focus on are all about supporting energy, the mitochondria and also helping support a healthy immune system. Typical issues on the medial end of things when this resilience type gets out of balance include chronic low energy, chronic fatigue syndrome, chronic Lyme, fibromyalgia and immune dysregulation as well as MCAS (mast cell activation syndrome) and autoimmune disorders.

- D Ribose: 5g per day. This is sugar that is used to help support mitochondrial function
- Acetyl L-carnitine: 500mg three times per day. Another nutrient needed to help support mitochondrial function.
- Fat soluble B-complex vitamin: 1–2 tablets per day
- Liposomal or S-acetyl glutathione. As we learned about in the food chapter, glutathione is the body's master antioxidant and is super-important for your cellular energy. Since it is hard to get a very high amount from foods alone, if you are already in the fatigued category and require a 'treatment' dose as opposed to a preventative dose, or you have tried to max out your diet already, I recommend adding a supplement of absorbable glutathione, which must say 'liposomal' if it is one taken by mouth or be in a newer form called S-acetyl glutathione, since ones that are not of this type are not well absorbed when taken by mouth as a pill. Generally, the dose for

fatigue and immune support is 600mg one to three times per day of liposomal, or 200mg/day and higher for the S-acetyl form. Milk thistle, which has the active ingredient silymarin, can also help boost glutathione levels and prevent depletion, so you can take this in addition to the liposomal glutathione to double the impact.

- Medicinal mushrooms. Normally I use a combination of a few medicinal mushroom extracts which have immune-system and energy-regulating properties and normally includes cordyceps and reishi as well as possibly others such as sun blaze, chaga, maitake, shiitake. I tend to use more than one type of mushroom for the potential herbal synergy effect rather than just one by itself, although they can also be used on their own too. There are many cheap mushroom powders online, but for this supplement it is important to choose a high-quality brand backed by a solid scientific formulation, since there is such a wide variation in the cheap versions versus the more expensive brands in terms of active ingredient content in the mushroom powder and hence effect. The dosage will vary depending on the formulation.

- Alpha lipoic acid: 600–1,800 mg per day may help with pain-related symptoms (e.g. fibromyalgia and nerve or 'neuro-' pain caused by a wide variety of illnesses such as Type 2 diabetes among many others) although it doesn't seem to work for everyone. It is quite a safe supplement.

- Co-enzyme Q10 in its ubiquinol form. People who suffer with chronic fatigue syndrome, for example, have been shown to have lower CoQ levels. CoQ10 is integral to energy production in our mitochondria.

- Phosphatidylcholine. One of the substances that makes up the cell membranes, it also may help with fatigue and brain fog.

- American ginseng (tired but wired) or panax ginseng (if just tired/ exhausted). These herbs have been shown to reduce fatigue.

- Pyrroloquinoline quinone (PQQ). This is a functional nutrient that in animal studies has shown to help with energy and aspects of brain and mental function. I use it in my patients with chronic fatigue combined with other nutrients.

WOUND-UP WARRIOR

Wound-up warriors need extra support calming down the nervous system and brain to return to a calm, cool and collected baseline so that they don't live constantly in a state of high chronic stress and 'hyperarousal' which depletes their resilience. These are in addition to magnesium (which is essential for reducing body noise and gets depleted with stress and 'wound-up' states), CBD and ashwagandha especially from the general list.

- L-theanine: This is a calming amino acid that is very safe. You can take 200mg per dose, up to three times a day, for anxiety but start with once a day in the evening.
- Inositol. Inositol is a supplement that is useful if you are prone to feeling panicky, on edge and have difficulty winding down. In one study, it was as effective as the leading drug treatment for panic disorder, a very severe form of anxiety, but with fewer side effects. So it can be extremely powerful even though it is 'natural'. The general dose is 3–5g up to twice a day. Decrease the dose if you experience any upset stomach or nausea, which can be a side effect especially at higher doses.
- Passionflower tablets or tincture, taken in the evening.
- 50mg tryptophan an hour or so before bed. This is a calming amino acid again that may help with winding down and reducing anxiety in the evening and before sleep/overnight to support better-sleep quality.

Tip: Add a few drops of Reishi tincture or CBD oil to your espresso for a more balanced caffeine boost with less jitters or crashing if you can't think of parting ways with coffee completely yet.

MOODY WARRIOR

Moody warriors need support with mood balance most of all, especially in times of higher stress.

- SAM-e stands for s-adenosylmethionine. The starting dose is around 400mg a day but sometimes higher. It is a chemical our bodies make from an amino acid, methionine, which is highest in animal-based foods such as eggs, chicken, beef and dairy. So if you are mainly dairy free and plant-based or vegan, you may not be getting much of this precursor from the diet. SAM-e is important because it helps regulate many essential cell functions, including brain-chemical balance related to mood, and many small studies have shown a positive effect on depression from supplementing with SAM-e. Generally, you should look for a brand that has individual blister packs for each tablet since it degrades easily. This is one you want to check with your doctor first too, to make sure it is right for you, especially if you are taking a higher dose.
- Vitamin B12. To make SAM-e, you also need Vitamin B12, so supplementing extra B12 even if your levels are in the 'normal' range may be helpful.
- Saffron. A number of studies have shown that saffron has similar properties to many antidepressant drugs used to treat depression and it has been used to treat different types of depression including post-partum depression in women with positive results. The dose generally is 15mg twice a day.
- Curcumin is the most well-researched active component of the turmeric root and is a potent anti-inflammatory in the brain and body. It has positive effects on the immune system's functioning and improving neuroplasticity and even the HPA stress-response axis between the brain and body, and reduces cortisol levels. It is often known best for its effects on joint pain, but it may also help with positive mood and mild depression with fewer side effects than antidepressant drugs according to some small studies. The positive mood effects may be even better when combined with saffron due to a possible synergy effect that is often seen in botanical medicine. Curcumin and its brain anti-inflammatory effects also makes sense in supporting mood because we know now that depression, at least in many people,

has a neuroinflammatory component. Ideally, choosing a highly absorbable form of curcumin reduces the dose needed to get a significant effect, since this nutrient is poorly absorbed on its own when taken by mouth. Dosage is 500mg twice a day.

- St John's Wort. This herbal stacks up well against antidepressant drugs for mild to moderate depression but with fewer side effects. The only downside is that it can interact with loads of medications, so if you take other medications, you need to check with your doctor to make sure this is a safe option for you. The other important point is that because there are so many sub-par products for St John's Wort out there, you should look for what's called a standardized formula with a known amount of the active herbal compound that has been measured accurately and use a trusted research-tested brand to get the best effect. The effects generally take about two months of taking it daily to kick in. The dose is generally 300mg three times a day of a standardized extract product.

SCATTERED WARRIOR

For scattered warriors, it's all about supporting brain focus, concentration and memory.

- American ginseng. This is a less 'anxiety-provoking' variety of the ginseng and, when combined with high-dose DHA and omega-3 fatty acids, may help improve focus. DHA is particularly important for scattered warriors, from krill or small fatty fish supplement-based sources. There are also a few algae (vegan friendly!) DHA sources if you are a scattered warrior and also a strict vegan.
- Huperzine A. This is an extract from Chinese club moss with medicinal properties for brain health and has been shown to reduce cognitive deficits in animal models. General dosage is 200mcg a day.
- Exogenous ketones are the only way to get the body to make more of the brain-protective ketone bodies that come with a low-carb diet, while still allowing you to have more diet flexibility

with the amount of healthy carbs you eat, e.g. potentially up to around 80 or 90 grams of carbs versus 20 grams a day. These are taken as a supplement three times a day. Be sure to check labels to ensure the only ingredient is the ketones, as many of these supplements also contain stimulants and other things you don't necessarily want or need or that can result in side effects.

WOMEN'S HEALTH SUPPORT

If you have specific issues related to women's health, following the above recommendations can make a significant difference because the supplements most helpful for everyone and then for your type can help many women's health symptoms too. For example, adding adaptogens may help you manage your stress response and regulate stress hormones better, which may be helpful in oestrogen excess issues where you may have too much oestrogen relative to progesterone in the second half of your menstrual cycle, leading to worse PMS, more painful or heavier periods. Magnesium, a supplement most people can benefit from, also helps with women's health issues such as PMS anxiety and period pain. Vitamin D helps not only regulate bone health but also is involved in ovulation and blood-sugar balance, which can get out of whack if you have PCOS. Normally, your type will also influence your women's health too, especially when you get out of balance. Moody warriors may be most prone to getting PMDD, which is a more severe form of PMS in terms of mood symptoms. The suggestions for your type may also help with moodiness before your period too. Wound-up warriors are most likely to have anxiety-type PMS, which can be reduced by following the wound-up warrior suggestions, and so on. In addition to this, an herb called chasteberry may also be helpful if you suffer from PMS or anovulatory cycles (when you don't ovulate or release an egg) due to chronic stress affecting the hypothalamus, since chasteberry may also promote ovulation by decreasing excess of another hormone called prolactin and also supporting progesterone, the hormone we need enough of to balance oestrogen.

Karen, forty-seven, came to see me to help her with what she described as women's health symptoms. When we sat down and dug into what her symptoms were, she explained that although she had always been 'high strung', it seemed that since her periods had become less regular the low-grade anxiety and sleep issues that she had managed to sort of ignore and 'get on with it' for years were becoming quite unbearable. She also felt more irritable at the slightest thing and was beginning to experience hot flushes and palpitations. She had been to see her GP who suggested, vaguely, exercise and meditation as first steps. So she then tried every form of meditation under the sun and diligently went for almost an hour's brisk walk each day. Although these things had some benefit, she was still feeling miserable and not in control of her symptoms, not to mention needing to rely on multiple cups of coffee due to her daytime fatigue after many restless nights. She was quite certain she did not want to go on HRT, even body-identical HRT (which I use with many patients and is the lowest-risk type of HRT, where you take hormones that are identical to your own rather than synthetic). However, her quality of life was so affected that she needed to do something, and fast. Based on her resilience type of wound-up warrior, we put her on a comprehensive resilience programme focused on supporting her transition into menopause. As part of her plan, we initiated a number of botanicals and supplements, including medicinal cannabis, ashwagandha, L-theanine and inositol, and sleep-support herbals as well as slow-release melatonin. We also added extra magnesium and omega-3s from krill in pill form on top of a diet high in these nutrients. For morning energy, we let her keep one cup of organic 'full-caf' coffee but added a tincture of mushroom and Siberian ginseng to help her maintain her energy without needing additional caffeine throughout the day. In three months, she was starting to feel like her old self again, and although she still had some perimenopausal symptoms, they were entirely manageable and no longer ruining her life.

So supplements can really help make a significant difference to resilience, even though they are not a magical quick cure-all. When combined together with food, mind–body practices and power plants, they can offer quicker gains and help support the brain and body in areas we may be struggling with due to a combination of genes and environment. No one is perfectly balanced in all areas. The trick is knowing what you are buying, how to combine things best for your type and situation – which you now know how to do, so you can get started with confidence. If you want to target a specific medical issue, get expert advice too before spending a fortune in the supplement aisle trying to DIY it.

CHAPTER 6

THE POWER PLANTS FOR RESILIENCE (CANNABINOIDS AND PSYCHEDELICS)

Tom came to see me with a long list of medical issues. His problems started off with anxiety as a teenager, then in his twenties he struggled with low mood and sleep, although he never saw a doctor and just 'got on with it'. That was until he had a skiing accident that left him with chronic back pain and things got a lot worse. He had to take strong pain-killers to help him get through the day, although he felt that they worsened his mood and made him feel 'not himself'. Tom was on a long list of medications that he wasn't sure were all that helpful and he suspected they were causing significant side effects. We decided to try medical cannabis to help him with his anxiety, mood and pain as well as help him get a deeper sleep. He also eventually wanted to wean down his pain and sleeping pills, which is another thing medical cannabis can help with. We started very slowly and over a six-month period his anxiety lessened, his daytime pain improved and he began to sleep better. His mood got better and because his pain was better controlled, he was able to start doing more exercise again, the one thing that he used to rely on to help him feel happier before his accident. He stopped his sleeping pill and his daily opioid painkillers completely and decreased his dose of some of the other medications. He felt clearer-headed, calmer and happier than he had in many years. He had always been scared of 'doing drugs', so the fact that medical cannabis had helped him achieve his new level of resilience and wellbeing was a huge surprise to him. Even though it wasn't a permanent cure for his problems, he felt like it had given him his life back.

Tom is a great example of someone whose seemingly unrelated and chronic issues can be helped by the use of what I like to call the 'power plants'. These get their own chapter in *The Resilience Blueprint* because, when used in the right hands in the right way, they are, as a group, among the most powerful tools out there for resilience.

Power plants are potent and they must be used responsibly and with caution and care, especially the ones that alter consciousness and change our state. However, these are tools that have been used in different cultures around the world since ancient times to help reduce suffering and to facilitate personal transformation and healing. Many of the power plants were considered sacred by the cultures that utilized them, and still are. However, in the last century they have also been misunderstood, maligned and feared, and only very recently have started to regain their place as respectable tools that could be used as modern medicines, because they do things modern pharma drugs can't. Those who utilized many of the power plants until recently (and still even now) did so in secret, because many of these compounds were and still are illegal in many places. But the resilience secrets they hold are beginning to be told again by the next generation of scientists finally allowed to study them once again, bringing more evidence to the transformations I have witnessed in some of my patients over the years who stepped outside the medical model to use these tools for their healing journeys.

The Cannabis Sativa Plant

The cannabis sativa plant is a treasure trove of active plant compounds that have powerful wellness and medicinal uses for enhancing resilience. After prohibition of this plant in many parts of the world in the twentieth century, largely due to politics rather than scientific reasons, medicine and research scientists are finally starting to catch up, discovering the superpowers of this plant. I have been using medical cannabis in the treatment of difficult-to-treat complex chronic conditions ranging from pain to anxiety for years, first in Canada and more recently since it became a legal medicine again in the UK, where I now practise. It's a resilience showstopper when used correctly.

Many people are now utilizing and incorporating plant compounds from the cannabis plant into their wellness regimens using over-the-counter CBD hemp varieties of the plant (which you can get legally in health shops and online). This can work quite well for things like stress and related symptoms since CBD is biologically active no matter whether it comes from a prescription medical cannabis product or a hemp variety you can buy yourself, as long as it is a good-quality product. In my medical practice, I also use prescription medical cannabis containing THC. THC you may know as the plant chemical that in large amounts can make you feel 'high' but, used in smaller amounts, and combined with CBD, it has incredible medicinal effects too when used correctly. Notice I say 'when used correctly' because when people overuse THC, it can actually cause issues with resilience – like more anxiety, for example – if you overshoot your very individual sweet spot. Smoking cannabis also burns the plant material, which may produce inflammatory compounds: also not so good for resilience, which is why I don't advocate smoking it for wellbeing or medical purposes. Medical cannabis containing THC has been life-changing for so many of my patients in helping to relieve very difficult-to-treat symptoms and dramatically improving their quality of life and hence their resilience potential.

When I trained as a medical doctor years ago, we were taught that cannabis was a dangerous, highly addictive drug of abuse, a 'gateway' drug to 'hard-drug' use and spiralling into a life-destroying addiction. No one knew or at least talked about the difference between CBD and THC, different strains, or that the cannabis plant has hundreds of bioactive plant compounds with wellbeing and medical potential. Over a decade later, having used cannabis to treat thousands of people and mentored many of my doctor colleagues in this art, since it's not quite as simple as prescribing someone a pill, one of my favourite sayings is that cannabis can indeed be a gateway drug: a gateway to meditation, resilience and improved quality of life!

Our Endocannabinoid System

Cannabinoids are powerful natural molecules for creating change in so many different aspects of wellbeing, health and resilience, as well as helping enhance life experience for many people. The reason cannabinoids are so helpful is because they work within our natural endocannabinoid system, or ECS for short, which we learned about in Part One. It's part of our resilience biology because its function is to help bring balance in brain and body, or homeostasis, and it helps regulate everything from our sleep–wake cycles to our mood and pain response.

This explains why medical cannabis and CBD seem to help with so many diverse and seemingly unrelated issues, symptoms and conditions.

There are well over a hundred cannabinoids, including CBD and THC, and although we know the most about CBD and THC, many of the other 'minor cannabinoids' have actions in our brain and body too and have medicinal value. In addition to all of the cannabinoids, there are also other bioactive plant-chemical groups in the plant, called terpenoids and flavonoids. All of these plant compounds work together in a plant cocktail known as herbal synergy or the 'entourage effect', to help fight inflammation, reduce stress, ease anxiety and sleep issues, help regulate immune function and various other processes like pain perception and supporting brain health.

So no matter what resilience type you are, the cannabis sativa plant likely has something interesting to offer you as a wellbeing tool when used correctly. Because cannabinoids have such a powerful effect, especially THC in terms of its psychotropic effects, too much THC can be a negative too. This is often the case with too much high-THC, low-CBD recreational-use cannabis used on a regular basis, when it can start to cause more imbalances rather than help them. For example, wound-up warriors who use too much THC should beware of 'rebound anxiety'. Too much THC daily for exhausted warriors may also worsen fatigue too, as opposed to micro or small amounts of THC combined with CBD that may improve stress, anxiety and fatigue. Stress and anxiety are actually the number-one reason people try to keep using a full-spectrum CBD product, which tends to be extremely effective and well tolerated, so it's a go-to for wound-up warriors, especially when you use a product with minor cannabinoids like CBN, cannabinol, which many people find both calming and useful for chronic pain, and calming terpenes like myrcene. Emerging research is showing that CBG, or cannabigerol, is another minor cannabinoid that in addition to its anti-tumour and anti-microbial properties may also be helpful for calming anxiety (wound-up warriors!).

For moody and exhausted warriors, you want to look out for varieties of cannabis that are labelled as 'sativa'-dominant and rich in terpenes like limonene and pinene. For example, when I treat patients with chronic fatigue syndrome or moody types who have trouble 'activating' in the morning, a very small dose of vaporized medical cannabis with one of these 'energizing' strains can help give them the energy to start their day well and help shift them out of a low mood faster.

Many people with ADHD symptoms also feel better and more able to focus and concentrate when they use a 'microdose' of THC containing cannabis (where legal) in the morning. A microdose is a bit of a vague term when it comes to cannabis, but generally it means a dose of THC below the level which would cause feelings of impairment or feeling 'high'. This may be most relevant for scattered warriors, who tend to struggle with focus. This is something I have found for years treating patients with medical cannabis who often have ADHD as well as anxiety or sleep problems or another additional reason to try medical cannabis. CBD may also help with the anxiety that many scattered warriors can experience because of mental overwhelm they can experience.

MEDICAL CANNABIS

In the UK, medical cannabis was made legal in 2018 and is now available as a prescribed medicine. When the law first changed, I had just moved back to the UK and became involved in training the first medical doctors in how to prescribe medical cannabis. Medical cannabis was something I had been using for years in Canada and was already a legal medicine in Israel and many parts of the US as well as in Australia. We know that cultures across the globe successfully used cannabis for medical reasons throughout history to significant effect. The research is finally catching up now that it is again legal to research and prescribe cannabis as a medicine in many parts of the world. We are rediscovering its many benefits for maintaining health and resilience and also fighting disease. THC, when used in medical cannabis, usually in low doses as part of a whole plant extract, it is highly beneficial for conditions such as chronic pain, muscle spasm and helping control symptoms in conditions such as multiple sclerosis, insomnia and nausea and vomiting as a side effect of chemotherapy, among others. Preliminary research shows that THC in ultra-low doses or microdoses taken daily may also help memory, and may be useful for diseases of brain ageing in healthy older adults as part of a preventative strategy. Microdosing THC from the cannabis plant as well as other psychotropic compounds for well-being and resilience is a practice that is gaining popularity and, very recently, being studied in formal medical research settings. Microdosing is no longer just for the hippies, but we are still at the early stages of research to fully understand all of its potential effects and benefits.

For exhausted warriors, cannabis and CBD can come in handy in multiple ways too. A medical cannabis product with THC (where legal) can help alleviate pain and improve sleep before bed. A hemp-based full-spectrum CBD product may also help with inflammation, taken either orally or transdermally (through the skin), and can be combined with other energy-rescue botanicals and supplements (see the supplements chapter, page 141). If you are trying to avoid alcohol and need another social tool to help with social anxiety or moodiness which can create barriers to getting out socially, some people find (where legal) that small amounts of cannabis can be used as a healthier alternative to alcohol for socializing.

How to Use The Cannabis Plant for Your Type

For all types, generally the safest way to start for most people is with a hemp-based full-spectrum CBD product that may have helpful effects on reducing stress and inflammation as well as having neuroprotective properties as part of a supplement wellbeing 'stack'. CBD hemp-derived 'full-spectrum' products still contain tiny amounts of minor cannabinoids and other plant chemicals that tend to contribute to the wellbeing benefits, including a 'microdose' amount of THC, still well under the legal limit and never enough to make you feel impaired. Most people take this as an oil or tincture by mouth (2–3 times a day), or now there are newer longer-acting ways to take it too, such as in transdermal patches that you change every two to three days.

Resilience Type	Cannabinoids of interest	Terpenes	Strains/chemovars
Wound-up	CBD, THC in a 'microdose' amount (too much can cause anxiety), CBN, CBG	myrcene, linalool	strains marked as 'indicas' for evening or hybrids for daytime
Moody	CBD, THC in micro/small doses, THCV (may help with food cravings)	limonene, terpinolene	strains marked as 'sativas' especially for mornings or hybrids.
Exhausted	CBD, THC in micro/small doses, THCA, CBN (for night-time/evening)	limonene, alpha pinene	strains marked as 'sativas' especially for daytime to reduce fatigue
Scattered	CBD, small or micro doses of THC also may be helpful for focus in ADHD and in cognitive function in older adults	alpha pinene	balanced strains, e.g. hybrids

Cannabinoids for Women's Health Resilience

An entire chapter in my last book, *The CBD Bible*, was devoted to this topic and since then we have discovered more about how many women's health conditions may be helped by cannabinoids. Generally, starting with a full-spectrum CBD product is the best way to go. However, for severe period pain or pain from endometriosis, a condition where uterine lining grows outside the womb where it shouldn't, creating pain and problems, THC containing medical cannabis can effectively treat pain and reduce the need for opioid pain-killers, while also improving feelings of wellbeing and quality of life. Perimenopausal symptoms are another area where CBD and medical cannabis are of great value for coping with symptoms, either on their own or combined with body-identical HRT and other integrative medicine strategies.

Therapeutic Psychedelics

In addition to cannabinoids, there are multiple other plant medicines and psychoactive molecules which are now being investigated and used as 'new medicines' in the mainstream medical sense, although most of these compounds are not new at all. Most have been legally prohibited for many decades, although before the twentieth century many were used widely for healing in many cultures. Their ban, like cannabis, has been largely due to political reasons rather than scientific ones, since as a group of drugs they have very low addictive potential. However, they are now coming back into mainstream medicine as fast-acting therapeutics for many mental-health conditions because of their incredible potential to change the brain in ways that current drug therapies cannot. I believe these compounds are going to radically change mental-health care as we know it for the better in the next decade.

Until recently and even now, any compound, whether from a plant or lab, that can alter someone's state of consciousness has been met with suspicion and fear, especially in the medical community. Like cannabis before it, doctors have a hard time wrapping their heads around the idea that using previously illegal compounds that we were taught were highly dangerous in medical school and could send everyone 'crazy' even after one use are now the most promising new medicines for conditions where western medicine is failing, namely in mental health, chronic complex conditions and pain. However, just like with cannabis, education and irrefutable emerging research is changing this bit by bit.

Psychedelic-assisted psychotherapy, an emerging mainstream medical therapy gaining wider acceptance due to a growing research base, as well as the use of these compounds in traditional ceremonies with an experienced traditional healer (known often as a shaman) are, in my view, two of the most powerful ways to harness a resilient temperament. This is especially true if you have found cultivating these traits very difficult in the past using other approaches alone. The key is having a safe, therapeutic environment and guide, since without these elements, healing and personal development are far less likely and the risks of purely recreational non-intentional use are much higher, especially for certain substances. However, in the right setting, these psychedelic experiences and journeys inwards represent an opportunity to gain a huge degree of self-insight and inner knowing in a relatively short period of time, especially when the experience is integrated and processed with a guide or therapist familiar with this work so that the changes can be more lasting and meaningful. I had one patient who had suffered from depression and addiction and had been to rehab multiple times but kept relapsing. Her depression was also resistant to treatment with multiple medications. We also know that depression, trauma and addiction often go hand in hand. She was really suffering and had spent a fortune on therapy. She decided on her own to go to South America to an intensive ayahuasca retreat centre that specialized in addictions. She spent a month preparing for the trip, changing her diet and meditating, and then another month at the retreat centre which included multiple doses of ayahuasca taken in a monitored group setting plus time for integrating the experiences and rest along with simple, healthy food and no access to alcohol or recreational substances. She returned from her trip without cravings for alcohol, significant improvement in her mood and has remained sober ever since. She kept going to NA meetings and seeing her therapist to maintain her remission, but the turning point in her journey was her therapeutic psychedelics experience. She decided to retrain as a therapist and now helps other people integrate similar therapeutic psychedelic experiences.

Most of these experiences are done either overseas in traditional ceremonies or illegally 'underground' in places like Canada, the US and the UK. I have been privileged that my patients have shared many such experiences with me over the years and felt they could include me in their journey. Usually, I have been the only doctor they had ever felt comfortable disclosing these experiences to. I have met patients who have been effectively 'cured' or at least put into long-term remission from conditions ranging from chronic fatigue syndrome to addictions and treatment-resistant depression by incorporating the therapeutic use of these compounds into their healing journey. In all cases, they had failed with traditional western medicine treatments and drugs, and before they discovered psychedelics had reached a point of hopelessness. Their experiences were nothing short of miraculous to them. In other cases, people noticed incremental improvements in similar difficult-to-treat symptoms although not as radical 'cure' results, and they continued to use them regularly (ranging from every few months to once a year) to maintain their health.

As with cannabinoid, or cannabis medicines, many of these compounds traditionally are still used in 'whole-plant' form or by combining multiple plants together. However, all of the plant medicines have known psychoactive compounds that have been isolated and we understand their effects, at least on a preliminary level. We still have a lot to learn though about them, since the research 'catch-up' is happening after a long ban on studying them.

I have also spent extensive time in various alternative communities and experienced the way that these substances are worked with first hand, just as I have seen with cannabis. I have seen how transformational they can be in the right hands, context, safe settings and, ideally, accompanied by integration and reflection work before and after the experience. When I first encountered the use of these substances, on my travels, my initial reaction as a trained medical doctor who had never used psychedelics recreationally (much like with cannabis!) was scepticism and even fear. However, through personal and professional experience I have come to understand the important role these compounds can play in healing and personal development. The fact that one of these molecules, psilocybin, from 'magic mushrooms', is now a bona-fide FDA-approved breakthrough drug is proof that the attitudes in mainstream medicine are changing. This section could be an entire book, but hopefully this will serve as a brief introduction to some of the 'newest' in terms of western medicine's view (or rather oldest, in terms of their rich traditional use history!) tools for resilience human beings have known for thousands of years.

In the area of mental health and brain resilience particularly, the emerging research on psychedelic medicines is the most exciting development in mental health for many decades, since current drug therapies are often ineffective, and none offer a cure for chronic conditions like major depression. Via multiple brain mechanisms that enhance novel thinking and brain flexibility, psychedelic molecules can also help people to recover from trauma, PTSD, addiction and heal severe chronic 'whole body and brain pain' conditions when other methods fail. They can also improve mental wellbeing and a sense of inner peace for people with terminal cancer. There is also emerging evidence that psychedelic medicines may work on the brain's immune system and reduce neuroinflammation, which has been implicated in conditions ranging from depression and chronic Lyme to Alzheimer's dementia. The biological effects we are discovering now that the research ban has been lifted in places like the US, Canada and the UK can help explain the science behind the numerous anecdotal reports of dramatic healing experiences people experience after using these substances.

I am including therapeutic psychedelics in the power plants chapter in this book on resilience because I truly believe from my clinical experience, as well as where the research is going, that this group of compounds is one of the most powerful resilience medicines out there. That is, when done in a legal, safe and therapeutic environment. The number of places where this is becoming possible in a legal medical or wellness environment is growing all the time. It is now possible if you live in the UK to go on legal psilocybin retreats in the Netherlands, only a short flight away. More 'normal' people who have never 'done drugs' go on retreats to help them overcome a health issue or just break out of a career or personal life rut, recover from burnout or simply to further their personal growth and resilience.

Set and Setting

The impact of psychedelic experiences and journeys on wellbeing and health conditions has a lot to do with something known as 'set and setting'. 'Set', short for 'mindset', refers to your state of mind and the mental preparation you do days and even a few weeks before taking the substance. Generally it involves ways to create a positive, relaxed state of mind leading up to the experience. This may involve a relaxation practice, time in nature, listening to music and journalling. It also involves exploring and talking about any fears, concerns or doubts about what your experience might 'be like' and what you want to get out of it. The experience itself is done in a therapeutic environment, with a trained facilitator, therapist or shaman/healer (in traditional-use ceremonies where legal).

'Setting' means the physical environment or setting where you will have your psychedelic experience. In a medical setting here in the UK, this is a medical clinic set up to be as calm and relaxing as possible. Or, in some research studies now ongoing in the UK, it may even be in a retreat setting supervised by medical doctors and set in nature and may also involve music, singing or chanting and creating a safe space.

Even with the same substance, generally most people will say that no two experiences are exactly alike, because our brains are dynamic and constantly changing. Another thing about therapeutic psychedelics is that they can enhance your mindset or mental state – any mental state you happen to be in. What that means is that depending on factors like set and setting, how much you take and the state of mind you are in when you take a journey, the experience can vary from very joyful to sad, overwhelming or very scary at times and be very challenging. That doesn't mean they are bad. In fact, many people who use psychedelics for therapeutic reasons say that their most challenging 'trips' or 'journeys' have been the most profoundly important. These experiences transformed them in a positive way or provided a piece of deep insight that allowed them to heal. That is why an experienced guide in a therapeutic environment is so important. I have been a 'trip sitter' or guide in a harm-reduction capacity where people had chosen independently to go on a trip. (*Note, I do not give people illegal substances; this has been in a legal harm-reduction capacity only.*) I have also had the opportunity to be part of people's debrief and self-reflection or 'integration' after taking one of these substances, in a medical context as part of caring for them as a patient and hearing their story. I feel very lucky to have had these opportunities because many patients are using these substances as part of their wellbeing journeys 'under the radar' but don't feel comfortable disclosing them to their doctor. It has allowed me to gain first-hand insight into the effects of these substances on resilience and wellbeing, since these are not things you learn about in medical school!

All of this may sound quite 'woo woo', especially coming from a trained medical doctor, but these are 'experiential medicines.' Unlike conventional drugs, the therapeutic effect depends not just on the 'psychedelic' part but what happens after that: using the insights from these altered states to create new brain pathways via the well-proven concept of neuroplasticity. Just taking a dose of LSD or mushrooms without any intention or preparation in a 'party' environment may be fun for some (or possibly not!), but it is unlikely to have the transformative therapeutic effect we see with proper use of these power plants.

The Dark Side of Psychedelics

Like all powerful tools, psychedelic substances, whether they come from a plant or a lab, can also have a dark side. I have seen this personally over the years where these substances are used outside the medical model. I have seen 'shamans' taking advantage of participants in ways ranging from slightly inappropriate to outright abusive. I've also seen people who suffered from a mental health condition like bipolar overuse these substances or use them inappropriately, leading to a prolonged manic episode and breaks from reality which took them many months to recover from. In some cases, the signs that things were 'going wrong' were overlooked by their friends and community – in one instance, as a sign of Kundalini awakening rather than a manic episode where they were repeatedly putting themselves in extremely risky situations. I have also had friends who had placed themselves in the hands of 'shamans' who ended up assaulting them on retreats and instead of improving their issues, ended up creating more trauma instead. However scary that sounds, when used by experienced therapeutic practitioners in a legal setting, these substances can be incredibly transformative. It's also just not with psychedelics that bad things happen in the wellness world. They also occur in the yoga world too, with unsavoury 'swamis' taking advantage of students in the same ways, also something I have seen first-hand. It also doesn't mean traditional-use ceremonies are 'bad' and that these substances can only be beneficial (where legal of course) in the setting of a doctor's office or hospital, but the additional checks and balances when they are used by trained clinicians and doctors in a medical or at least legal therapeutic setting (like a medical ketamine clinic, or a legal retreat with trained professional therapists), for example – minimizes the risks. The emergence of psychedelic-therapist training programmes by reputable organizations is helping with this issue. These programmes are training facilitators who come from the healing professions but are not limited to doctors, since a medical degree is not necessary to provide excellent facilitation. Of course, only try these substances in a safe legal setting, not illegally on your own.

Specific Compounds and Plant Medicines

Some of the compounds below are now being used in psychedelic therapy settings with a medical doctor and trained psychotherapists. Others, such as plant medicines like ayahuasca, are still mainly used under the guidance of a non-medical experienced guide, traditional healer or shaman. As a group, when used responsibly, these compounds offer tremendous hope and potential for treatment-resistant medical conditions as well as offering potential for self-discovery and personal growth and essentially greater brain resilience. Each resilience type may benefit in different ways from these experiences (again, where safe and legal).

KETAMINE

Ketamine was initially developed in the 1960s as a painkiller and then used as an anaesthetic for surgery. In the last twenty years, ketamine has also become a promising treatment for chronic pain and, more recently, for treatment-resistant depression. It is thought to work as an antidepressant by rewiring/resetting brain networks involved in depression and creating new brain connections. In essence, it can restore some of the brain-resilience networks involved with mood and pain control. It works on chronic pain, for example, by changing how the brain processes pain in ways that other drugs like painkillers can't.[1] It tends to work more quickly, in a matter of hours, versus traditional antidepressants which take multiple weeks, if they work at all. Conventional antidepressants are also not good at treating the cognitive problems, like low motivation and the brain fog of depression even when they work for other symptoms. Ketamine seems to work better for all of these and, even though not widely used as first-line treatment, is considered a safe medication when used under medical guidance. It can also be used at the higher 'psychedelic' or more accurately, 'dissociative', doses combined with psychotherapy to produce lasting positive effects on mood.[2] Ketamine also works when other drugs like painkillers or conventional antidepressants have failed. It is generally given via an IV or as an injection to begin with, in a session that is supervised at a specialized medical clinic and followed by a therapy session with a trained psychotherapist to 'integrate' the session and get the most brain changes. The number of doses a patient will need and how often can vary quite a bit. Ketamine is also used as a nasal spray in smaller doses for treatment-resistant depression, which moody warriors are more likely to experience compared to the other types. Ketamine lozenges that you dissolve in the mouth or a liquid form you drink can also be used instead of IV to avoid the needles and are becoming more popular as we gain research about this method. The needle-free approach has been shown in one recent study to be effective and safe for treatment-resistant chronic pain.[3] In my patients who suffer with both mood and chronic pain issues who have 'tried everything', often the combination of medical cannabis and ketamine therapy completely changes their lives after years of suffering at a high level of disability and very low level of resilience. Ketamine therapies are currently available in the UK mainly in private clinics but not yet widely available on the NHS, although I suspect this will change in the future.

Mary came to see me for treatment-resistant depression. We had tried all the conventional medications and then added medical cannabis. While it helped with her sleep and her fibromyalgia pain, her depression was still stubborn to shift. We decided on ketamine therapy, and I referred her to my colleague who specializes in this treatment. She was a bit scared to try it, since she had never taken any psychedelics recreationally, but she was up for anything that would help her depression, which was preventing her from having relationships and a successful professional life. She responded within a few sessions and thankfully the treatment continued to work. She was able to move to more spaced-out maintenance doses and said it was the first time in her adult life that the black cloud of depression didn't rule her life. She felt more clear-headed and her brain 'just worked better'. Her fibromyalgia improved too. She was able to start a new relationship and landed a job she loved. Ketamine therapy essentially gave her a life again that depression had stolen from her, and she continued to use it alongside medical cannabis in low doses with great results.

LSD

LSD is short for d-lysergic acid diethylamide. It's a compound discovered by a researcher named Albert Hoffman in the 1940s by slightly changing a plant molecule found in nature in a type of fungus called 'ergot fungus'. So technically it's man-made but it does have plant medicine origins. In the 1950s and 1960s, LSD was used by mainstream medicine in psychotherapy. Over 1,000 medical research papers were published on its use in therapeutic settings to treat conditions ranging from addiction to depression with promising results before it was banned even for research use due to political reasons and a cultural backlash to the hippie movement. The fact that it actually has a researched use history got very well buried to the point where we definitely didn't learn about it in medical school. Similar to the cannabis plant's 'bad rep' history, when someone first told me about the LSD medical studies, I thought they were crazy.

This ban stalled research and medical use for over half a century and created a huge stigma against the molecule, especially in the medical community, more so than with any other psychedelic. Mainstream medicine and scientific research have restarted, however, and are currently investigating LSD in clinical trials to treat various conditions including headache disorders and mood disorders. Taking a psychedelic dose of LSD may also lead to a lift in mood for days afterwards for some people, which is why it is currently again under investigation for conditions such as depression and anxiety as it has become legal as a research molecule in many places once again (wound-up and moody warriors, watch this space!).

In more recent years, LSD has been a substance increasingly used as a self-development substance in extremely small or 'micro' quantities (even classic doses of LSD are already in the microgram range, so we are talking super-micro here). The definition of 'micro-dosing' for psychedelics is taking sub-perceptual (i.e. unnoticeable) amounts of the substance below the dose which changes the perception of reality or causes you to 'trip' or hallucinate, or anything close to this. In fact, if you notice any substantial change in perception, you have gone beyond a microdose into what's known as a low dose and would need to lower the dose further to get into the microdose range. Reasons people have tried microdosing in the non-medical context include help with mood, anxiety, focus and creative problem-solving abilities, to improve energy, enhance their EQ and generally feel happier in daily life. Some small recent studies have shown that, contrary to previous belief, microdosing is not a placebo and does have biological effects. I have had patients tell me about their experienced therapeutic benefit from microdosing on their own when nothing else worked for them. I can't wait for more research in this area to further explain the many 'case reports' I have witnessed, just like what happened with medical cannabis a few years ago, which brought it back into the realm of respectable medicine and its use in a legal medical context.

PSILOCYBIN (MAGIC MUSHROOMS)

Psilocybin is the psychotropic, meaning psychedelic, compound found in what is known as 'magic mushrooms', which are a group of fungi numbering over 180 species of different mushrooms found all over the world in nature. They are often found in farmer's fields where cows graze and most people pass them without knowing their psychedelic secret (note: they also look very similar to some very poisonous mushrooms so never go picking on your own!). These types of psychedelic mushrooms have a long history of spiritual and healing ritual use. More recently, psilocybin has been recognized for its medicinal value in mainstream medicine to treat a variety of conditions ranging from depression, anxiety and PTSD to cluster headaches and addiction, with promising early results and recent recognition by the USD FDA of psilocybin as a 'breakthrough-therapy' drug for depression.

Psilocybin is similar to the chemical make-up of serotonin, known as our 'happy brain hormone', and docks into these receptor sites in the brain. It causes changes in the brain's 'filtering' information system, quiets down parts of the brain including something called the default mode network, and may help the brain get out of stuck ruts involved in perpetuating chronic pain syndromes and depression, similarly to ketamine but by a different mechanism. Psilocybin is illegal in the UK currently outside of research. Magic mushrooms have been decriminalized in some jurisdictions such as in Colorado, USA. They are also legal in Brazil. In the Netherlands, psychoactive mushroom species available there classified as truffles, which are fully legal, have allowed legal therapeutic 'personal-growth' magic-mushroom wellness retreats to pop up. These are becoming increasingly popular with people in the UK and Europe as a legal and accessible tool for healing, personal growth and resilience.

AYAHUASCA

Ayahuasca is the name for a tea with psychedelic properties from the Upper Amazon in South America. It is typically made from plants containing the psychedelic compound DMT (N,N-Dimethyltryptamine) as well as other bioactive plant compounds that contribute to its effects in a brew. The active ingredient DMT acts on serotonin receptors in the brain. With ayahuasca, many people report a deeply spiritual experience which can range from terrifying to euphoric and may in turns alternate between these two extremes in the same session. Ayahuasca is also known for the 'purging' element, which can include intense nausea, vomiting, and diarrhoea. For these reasons, ayahuasca is not generally taken for fun or 'recreationally'. This tea has been used for centuries amongst the indigenous tribespeople of Amazonia for both shamanic and medicinal purposes, under the guidance of a traditional shaman, or healer, for both mental and physical issues in indigenous culture in a ceremonial ritual.

More recently, ayahuasca has become more popular in the west, outside of this traditional context. Ayahuasca retreats have become popular in places where it is legal, such as in many South American countries and also in Costa Rica, which is one of the most popular westerner destinations for legal ayuhuasca retreats, including for people from the UK. It also now exists quite widely in underground weekend-retreat-style ceremonies throughout many countries, including the UK, where many people seek out this plant for healing and personal-growth experiences. So far research into the tea has shown its promising therapeutic potential for use in medical settings in the treatment of depression and addictions, often where other conventional treatments have failed. Anecdotal reports of healing from very difficult-to-treat conditions such as addiction, depression, PTSD and even chronic fatigue syndrome have also been reported by participants, something I have heard from some of my own patients and people I have known personally over the years who have gone on ayahuasca retreats where they are legal. DMT is also currently being used in a medical-research setting in places including the UK, but is not yet available for patients.

SAN PEDRO

San Pedro is a cactus native to the Andes regions in South America. It contains mescaline, a psychedelic compound also found in other cacti such as the peyote cactus. Mescaline-containing plants have also been used for thousands of years in traditional healing ceremonies by different indigenous cultures. Sometimes, it is combined in multi-day ceremonies with ayahuasca in some places where both are legal. San Pedro is traditionally used on its own or with other plants in a ceremonial brew under the guidance of a trained traditional healer. It is legal in Peru, Ecuador and Bolivia, where many people travel for retreats. It's also known for its ability to enhance feelings of compassion and gratitude during the experience and has been used by indigenous peoples to treat conditions such as depression and PTSD. One Harvard study on regular ceremonial use of peyote, a very similar plant with the same active ingredient, showed a decrease in addiction with no negative neuropsychiatric (i.e. mood or thinking) problems from regular use in a native American population, who are allowed to use it legally in some US states.

MDMA-ASSISTED PSYCHOTHERAPY

MDMA is a man-made drug best known for its recreational use in club and rave culture. However, it was first used in a medicinal context to enhance the benefits of psychotherapy in the 1970s as a respectable, though still experimental, treatment option. That was before it was banned in the US due to the rise of its recreational use in the 1980s, which stopped research studies until recently. It creates an experience of euphoria (i.e. intense joy), connectedness, empathy and energy. MDMA is now a promising therapy for PTSD, social anxiety and alcohol-use disorder, and possibly as a treatment alongside psychotherapy to treat depression, all under medical use. I once met a guy who relayed his very interesting experience with MDMA somewhere in the grey zone between recreational and therapeutic use. This often happens after I tell people the sort of medicine I do. When he was nineteen, he and his sister, who was two years older, had always had a difficult relationship, were at loggerheads again and their parents desperately wanted them to get along better. So they booked the whole family on a festival weekend and took MDMA together as a family bonding experience. Apparently, this weekend of bonding under the influence did improve the sibling relationship and the change seemed to stick. He said he was able to feel more empathy for his sister and they managed to get through the weekend without a major row for the first time in the history of family vacations since he could remember. Possibly the most unconventional parenting strategy I have ever heard, that's for sure (although of course I don't recommend illegal use of MDMA!).

That is a whirlwind tour of the power plants. Even if you are not in a position to venture into the deep end of power-plant territory yourself, I hope you may have a more open mind towards some of the previously controversial plants and substances and their resilience potential now that you understand a bit more about what they do. Even if you just use a CBD product, you are already set to benefit from 'power plant-lite'.

CHAPTER 7

MIND–BODY RESILIENCE

'But I already know how to relax,' Christie told me, when I let her know that we would be starting our stress-management work together with relaxation training. She protested that she went to a pre-work power-yoga class three days a week and each evening would unwind with Netflix and a single glass of wine. She was fit and healthy, and considered herself a relaxation pro. She worked in finance in the City, and on the surface life was great. However, as a wound-up warrior she was showing all the signs that her resilience was in troubled waters: the feeling like a lump in her throat that never seemed to go away lately, the shortness of breath episodes (after a fully normal heart and lung health check) and the trouble falling asleep and feeling unrested more mornings than not. It's not that the morning yoga class wasn't helping or that unwinding with a bit of TV was bad or wrong, but those things were just not activating the specific response in the brain and body to actually relax the nervous system on a deeper level. When Christie thought she was relaxing, her brain was still running the stress programme in the background below her level of conscious awareness. Even in her morning yoga class, the mental worry loops were still running rampant as she downward-dogged and saluted the sun for almost an hour.

If the mind is still running in worry loops and constant mental chatter, even if you're technically 'relaxing', it's not registering as relaxation in the brain sense. This kind of surface relaxation state is what twentieth-century yogi Swami Satyananda Saraswati called 'sensory distractions' rather than what is truly, deeply relaxing for your nervous system. This doesn't mean your yoga class is no good, but if your mind is still whirring, that class is not doing what you think it is. This is why many people still feel chronically stressed, overwhelmed or burned out even if they take 'time out to sit down and relax' on a regular basis. Your body may be lounging but the brain and breathing can be still 'jacked-up' on stress, not returning to a nice low-stimulation, low-stress state as our ancestors once did after an immediate threat had gone and things were safe again. The skill of deeply relaxing and 'winding down' the nervous system is something not taught in schools, or even to doctors. But the skill of learning to calm our nervous system on a regular basis is essential to opening the door to brain resilience in the face of the daily stress burden we face in modern life. We can learn how to turn on this resilience superpower by tuning in to what practice or practices may best suit our type and the resilience temperament traits we need to work on to help bring us back into balance.

Developing your mind–body resilience practice

Often when patients first come to see me, they are resistant to mind–body practices such as yoga or meditation. They want to focus on more 'tangible' things like their diet, supplements, medical cannabis and CBD, and often doing some functional-medicine tests to see what is out of balance from a very objective perspective. As previous chapters have explained, these all play an important role and patients love that they are very quantifiable or knowable, which our brains tend to like. Humans like to know when we are 'doing it right' and relate to metrics that demonstrate 'proof' of where things are at. However, I have found that mind–body skills and techniques are often the missing piece of the resilience jigsaw for my patients. I encourage both them and you to keep an open mind!

There are many different and often confusing terms when it comes to mind–body techniques: meditation, mindfulness, mind–body practices, contemplative practices, breathwork, yoga. I call them mind–body practices as a group, as what works for one person won't necessarily appeal to another. The key is to find what works best for you, and stick to it.

Mind—body practices enhance resilience by enhancing the ability of the brain to change itself. In the words of one group of researchers, these practices are like 'opening a window to brain plasticity'.[1] Plasticity means flexibility, and a flexible brain is a resilient one. Engaging in these practices also helps us access our natural RR, or relaxation response. As explained earlier, Netflix and a glass of wine doesn't cut it with the RR. We need a more active or deliberate kind of relaxation to rebalance a frazzled nervous system. That doesn't mean rest and relaxation watching a movie is bad; it's just not the same as doing a mind—body practice in terms of what it does on a brain level.

If you're new to mind—body practices, they can feel a bit daunting. They're a little more nebulous than taking a supplement or doing physical exercise. It can also feel harder to know if you are 'doing it right', which is very normal since it's a new skill for most of us.

Scattered warriors, for example, can tend to feel frustrated when they first start doing a mind—body practice because it can feel very hard to focus. The brain area called the parahippocampus, which helps prevent distraction, may be less engaged in scattered types, but it gets a workout and grows as you stick with a daily practice. Their minds may try to tell them to do it later when they have more time to 'get it right'.

Wound-up warriors may have more anxiety initially after starting their practice because of worrying that they didn't do it correctly or obsessing about doing it in perfect detail.

Moody warriors can often feel temporarily a bit more sad than before because they get more consciously aware of their moods.

Exhausted warriors may tend to start out strong but overdo it and end up feeling more tired, so then bin it altogether.

These are all totally normal reactions and temporary ones. If you are not sure when to start, the most perfect moment to start is the present one. The next-best moment is literally tomorrow. Really there is no future perfect time to start. Schedule your chosen practice with a timer set on a phone or watch or analogue timer and put it into your calendar. Keep continuing to practice through this mental doubt and discomfort, which should improve after one week of daily practice for most people, sometimes much sooner!

An effective mind–body practice need not be difficult or take up an hour a day to reap the huge resilience benefits. And remember those little DNA hats called telomeres that control how fast we age and the longer they are the better? Mind–body practices also lengthen your telomeres after just eight weeks, literally helping to slow down your cell-ageing process. Mind–body practices also help shut off stressful genes via a process called epigenetics. They promote growth of new brain cells and boost brain resilience via multiple pathways, even for total beginners in a matter of weeks. These practices also work by balancing those two arms of the ANS (autonomic or automatic nervous system from Part One). It's that powerful.

Finding your unique stress signature

Before we get into different mind–body practices and which type they may suit best, for every type the first introduction to your mind–body practice I feel should be learning how to 'diagnose' your body and brain's own 'stress signature'.

As we discovered in Part One, our inbuilt 'stress alarm system' in the brain has not quite fully adapted to modern life. The limbic system and HPA axis can get hypersensitive to stress and the areas of the brain that light up with the RR (relaxation response) haven't been exercised that much. This can mean the brain mistakes everyday daily events and small but stacked-up stressors like work deadlines, being late and even email alerts as actual threats to our safety or survival and sounds the alarm. We have trouble turning that alarm back off again.

Most people who have chronic stress and high cortisol often report not 'feeling particularly stressed' because the chronically stressed state becomes the brain's new normal, so we don't notice it any longer. It's like you no longer notice the alarm or block it out. It's the brain's way of trying to protect you, but the issue is that the effects are still there, lurking in the background. So the first step is discovering if that stress alarm is switched on in the background below the level of your conscious awareness.

This sneaky stress alarm going off in the background also explains the crazy stat that up to 90 per cent of visits to the GP are stress-related in some shape of form. Research proves that turning on your RR has helped people suffering from a diverse mix of diseases ranging from heart disease to diabetes as well as a host of mental-health and immune-health disorders, by helping turn off this alarm. Mind–body practices are still not taught by most doctors despite the huge body of evidence that they help rewire a stressed brain to a more resilient one. I have been teaching my patients simple techniques for over a decade. It generally takes as little as three to five minutes to teach a simple technique to someone. That is enough time generally so that they feel confident enough to go and try it at home and then report back after a week or two.

If we are not aware of what I like to call our stress signature, it is more difficult to know what the opposite of that stress feels like too, as you get more skilled at your mind–body practice, since you will have nothing consciously to act as a contrast. The 'stress signature' can be slightly different for each person. It may include body sensations such as a lump-in-the-throat feeling or tightness in the chest (that has been proven not be heart-problem related). It can even be a sensation that gets consciously buried for many years until you tune in to it in a relaxed state, such as chronic pelvic tension, something I have come across in my medical practice many times but that most doctors are totally unaware of. These stress markers relate back to, again, an imbalance between the SNS stress response arm and the PNS, but because the SNS does so many things, it can show up so differently. Whatever your signature is, once you find it you can start working on calming it before it ramps up and gets out of control and difficult to contain, using a mind–body technique for just a few minutes a day. This will help you stay more balanced and feel less bad stress over time and, ultimately, take your resilience to new levels.

Everyone has a different way that brain stress shows up for them and most of it is really subtle unless you know what to look for. Again, people don't consciously 'feel' the bad stress until things are really out of whack. This is because at those lower levels, unless we know how to tune in to our unique signs, the brain is really good at tuning it out so we can still function, although not at our best. For example, if you are a wound-up warrior, you may not feel it until you start having symptoms of physical anxiety, shortness of breath or even panic attacks. If you are an exhausted warrior, you may need three-day weekends where you feel you need to sleep all day to recover for the next week. For moody warriors, your stress response may be to withdraw and avoid everything and everyone or become super-irritable over the smallest thing. For scattered types, the sense of overwhelm can lead to whole days of zero productivity, paralysed with 'choice overwhelm' and procrastination because it feels impossible to know where to start anything and the harder you try to focus the more impossible it becomes, coupled with a sense of physical restlessness.

To become aware of how brain stress 'shows up' for you, you have to identify what unique combination of feelings and body sensations are your brain's way of telling you it is stressed out.

If you have chronic pain, for example, over time the nervous system can start to perceive even non-painful sensations as painful, through a process called 'neurological wind-up' where the brain gets hypersensitive to things like touch but also even things like loud noises and strong smells. These sensitivities can get worse, the more stress you are under. So if you do suffer with chronic pain, recognizing the subtler signs of this 'wind-up'/hypersensitivity before things spiral into a pain crisis is really useful for helping to manage not just your pain but also your brain-stress levels over time too.

Common Body Sensations of Stress

- Tightness in shoulders, throat, chest, neck or jaw
- Lump in throat
- Funny feeling in stomach or gut
- Dizziness, lightheadedness
- Sweating
- Feel heart beating fast

- Dry mouth
- Physical restlessness, feeling unable to sit still or needing to fidget, not able to stay comfortable sitting down while working, for example

Here are some less physical signs of stress to watch for:

- Feeling on edge
- Feeling mentally restless
- Feeling frustrated
- Feeling overwhelmed
- Feeling brain-foggy
- Feeling low
- Having a sense of dread
- Cravings for carbs, sugar or salty, fatty foods
- Feeling emotionally 'numb'

If you can't pin down a feeling but just get the general 'overwhelm' or 'exhausted' feeling, that's OK. Once you start tuning in, you may notice more specific signs of stress like tight jaw muscles or neck tension, for example. You can use the following one-minute breathing practice to help you tune in to your stress levels throughout the day and then calm them back down before it spirals.

The Quick Start Practice for All Types

If you are new to mind–body practices or meditation, it is extra-important to make your practice simple, fast and doable. This gives our brains a win every day for the least amount of mental effort so those feel-good chemicals keep coming and we stay motivated. The one-minute 'resilience-reset' practice can be integrated into even the most hectic of days. It lets us keep reminding our brains of the ruts it tends to fall into throughout the day, and catch it before things spiral out of control. You can create a one-minute 'resilience reset' out of many of the mind–body and meditation practices in this chapter, but to keep things simple for now, I am going to teach you one that works for every resilience type, as a place to start.

Again, the key is to keep reminding your brain each day how to access your relaxation response state more naturally and easily over time and set you up for more resilient days in normal, hectic life without thinking about it as you get 'unconsciously competent' at this skill over time.

Another way of thinking of this short one-minute practice is sort of like a brain reboot, similar to when your computer starts to run slowly and crash due to too many programs running in the background. Often it happens without you realizing it, eventually leading to a crash, or the 'wheel of death' on a Mac, as I like to call it, when your system stops responding. In order to make it run smoothly again, you have to close all the background tabs, do a complete restart and even, in some cases, more of a full-fledged back-to-factory settings reboot and clear your hard drive to make some space. When you start using these mini 'reboots' during the day to change your brain state, you are also building brain flexibility, one of the resilience temperament traits needed for all resilience types.

So even if you are feeling a bit too overwhelmed to read this entire chapter to find a more specific practice for your type right now, doing this one-minute breathing practice a few times each day is an incredible start. In fact, these few minutes of this practice alone over six to eight weeks may bring significant changes no matter what your type is. Then, when you feel ready to take the next step, you can add to your practice using the guides in this chapter based on your type. I chose a breath-focused practice for this reset because breath is the most direct way to access our parasympathetic nervous system and turn on our relaxation response for most people.

This is the practice I teach most to my patients in short visits, and I did this especially when I was in family practice and would only have five or ten minutes with each patient.

One-minute Relaxation Breath Exercise

Breathe all the air out first, then relax your belly and let it fill with air naturally without forcing anything, and both the lower ribs and the belly should move out. Then as you exhale, make a gentle *haaaa* sound and gently press your belly to your spine. Try to make your exhale at least twice as long as your inhale. Repeat for one minute. You can do this practice standing, sitting or lying, but the easiest way to learn how to engage the diaphragm is by starting lying down, to remove gravity as a factor, and then once you feel like you have got it, you can move on to trying it sitting at a desk and even standing if you are on the go.

I call this one- to two-minute RR breathing your 'resilience reset' because it helps move your nervous system into that calm state throughout the day, again and again, so toxic stress doesn't build up over a day to leave you feeling drained, fatigued and overwhelmed by day's end or feeling 'tired but wired' and then having trouble winding down for a restorative sleep. Try to do the practice at least three times a day and then again while you are in bed just before sleep. This only totals around five minutes a day, but will kickstart your resilience and build your confidence in your mind–body practice skills.

You can do an additional thirty seconds of this practice through-out the day if you notice signs of your 'stress signature', to help reset the stress levels before they build up.

The first step to change is becoming aware, and this can take time. So if you don't feel anything the first time you try this (or the first dozen times!), don't panic. The act of bringing your aware-ness into your body is a mind–body practice in itself that is already making your brain more resilient even if it feels like nothing is happening yet.

The next step is to take that awareness of that stress signature when you feel it coming on, and activate your relaxation response by using your chosen mind–body practice for your type or just start with the breathing practice above.

BREATHING PRACTICE CHEAT SHEET

Set a phone alert for a minimum of three times a day to remind you to do your breathing practice in the morning, noon and after dinner and before bed.

When you hear the alert, start your practice for one to three minutes.

Sit in a comfortable position, feet flat on the floor (or lying down if you are able and prefer it).

Close your eyes if you are able, but if not, simply do with eyes open or a lowered gaze to reduce distraction.

Start by exhaling all the air out of your lungs.

On the next inhale, gently feel the belly moving out as well as the lower ribs and picture in your mind your breathing muscle moving down and outwards in your chest, letting go of any tension in your abs.

Exhale slowly, making a gentle *haaaa* sound as you exhale. When you do this, you will notice your belly will gently naturally fall, the belly button moving back towards the spine (i.e. the belly should fall and contract slightly, but not forcefully).

How Even Long-time Yogis Can Have 'Stressed Brains'

At our wellness centre in Bali, we used brain-mapping analysis QEEG technology to see what is going on in the brain. Often, even people who have been practising physical yoga (and even meditation) daily for years would often have brain stress or hyperarousal patterns on the EEG. Oftentimes, these patterns were seen in people coming to the centre because of symptoms of stress, anxiety or moodiness despite their extensive daily practice. I have also had patients over the years who found that unless they did an entire hour of meditation twice a day, they could not handle the everyday stresses of life. It was so perplexing to them that their quite advanced practice 'wasn't translating' to less stress during their day. More than one such patient was also a meditation teacher (and a very good one at that). These people were experts at their technique, practised it faithfully and taught widely but still had a lot of suffering internally, often with low moods or anxiety. This often made them quite feel guilty because they thought this made them a yoga or meditation 'failure' or would activate their impostor syndrome.

Over the years living in conscious communities, I also found that many people with advanced yoga practices which they do for hours each day also still seemed deeply unhappy. How could this be so?

The first part of the answer, I think, has to do with the fact that people who have actively started a mind–body practice often do so because they have experienced stress, anxiety, depression or a similar issue and are on their healing journey, trying to find ways to bring more balance and happiness into their life. They are doing this more actively than someone who has not experienced such an issue with mood or mental wellbeing to the same degree. So even though they may still be suffering, they are likely better than they would have been without any practice.

However, the second part of my theory, based on the brain research on meditation, is that different techniques actually create slightly different brain states and develop different brain-resilience skills. So even if you are doing a practice each day but it's not the best fit for your type, you may be getting fewer benefits than expected.

In modern life, most of us want to take up one of these practices not for the pure sake of it, but to help us become more resilient, function better and feel happier.

When this is the goal, we want to choose something short, easy to do and somewhat tailored to our type.

Categorizing Meditation and Mind–body Practices

Researchers, scientists and even meditators themselves are still trying to agree on a classification or way of categorizing different mind–body practices and meditation types. The obvious reason why you'd want to do this is to see if a specific type or technique – for example, mindfulness – had unique effects on the brain. Or whether a technique seems to work really well for everyone to the same degree or just certain people or personality types (or resilience types). It would be great if this was a super-neat and tidy system where everyone fitted perfectly into a box of what practice would be ideal and complete for them. However, many of the studies on meditation combine techniques or define them differently, making it hard to establish clear trends or single out comparisons of one technique directly against another. We are all dynamic, complex, unique beings and in reality the systems that researchers have come up with so far to put different mind–body techniques into tidy 'bins' are still quite subjective, and the practices do overlap with each other in many instances. However, based on advanced brain imaging and EEG brain-signal studies, it does seem that some meditation techniques activate different neural, or brain, networks and work in different ways. Sort of like different 'brain skills', as I like to think of it. This is also likely why some techniques may work better for certain resilience types too. It is also important to note that in traditional eastern philosophical schools of thought and systems of meditation, many techniques are taught and combined alongside each other at different stages of training, and mastery is part of a many-years-long process. Just like we see in botanical (herbal) medicine, these techniques were likely 'synergistic', meaning they amplified the good effects of the other ones and helped build more resilient networks in the brain over time. This is often quite different from how we see meditation in the west. Mindfulness, for example, came from a traditional system and was just one technique that was taught to students. However, it has become highly successful as a stand-alone technique in the west to help with resilience in modern life. As a stand-alone, it can help with everything from reducing anxiety and chronic pain to having higher life and relationship satisfaction. Most people can benefit from doing just a few minutes of this practice each day, regardless of your type. If there is one simple meditation style that is good for every type, it's probably mindfulness.

I always get asked if doing any mind–body practice is better than none, even if it may not be the best one for your type. The answer is generally yes, as any technique done consistently should help the brain and mind become more resilient over time. However, by keeping your type in mind, it can really help to create a practice that is most beneficial for the least time investment each day. We will explore a few different techniques and the resilience types they may suit best, and which ones are good for everyone too.

Where to Start Based on Your Type

Most of my patients know or at least have heard that 'meditation' is a thing that is good for them, but most, even those who regularly attend yoga classes, do not know where to start or what practice is right for them. If you don't yet have a mind–body or meditation-type practice, this is a guide for where you can choose to begin, based on which technique may be most balancing for your type and also for the top resilience traits you feel you need to work on most.

This is a great way to figure out where to start with a short practice you can do each day for just a few minutes and gain mastery over. Later on, you may wish to combine a few techniques too, which is something I do myself and is helpful since it is rare that we are purely one type or need only type of skill. Combining a few practices together need not take a lot more time, but can be done in small chunks, such as one to two minutes per practice in a mini combo. This is something I often help my patients do too. It also helps build brain flexibility too, another of the top-ten resilience traits. There are many meditation videos, apps and tools available to learn each of these practices once you decide on one you'd like to practise.

Summary of Top Practices for Your Type

These are all detailed in this chapter in the following pages to show you exactly how to do it, this is just a handy summary.

Moody	Wound-up	Exhausted	Scattered
Loving kindness/ compassion meditations Gratitude practices such as Three Good Things and the Grateful Jar Activating moving meditation: Flying Goose Activating pranayamas (breathing) especially for the morning such as: bhastrika or kapalbhati, balancing breathing practices such as alternate-nostril breathing (nadi shodhana) Altered-states mind-body work through breath with guided holotropic breathwork, therapeutic psychedelics (where legal and appropriate for you)	Body noise body-focused relaxation practices such as PMR (progressive muscular relaxation) Mind noise: the Benson Technique Calming breaths such as the Healing Breath, Bee Breath	Yoga nidra Mindfulness Energizing breath: bhastrika Cleansing Breath: kapalbhati	Concentration meditation Mindfulness Focusing breath: ujjayi Balancing breath: nadi shodha

Mindfulness

- Resilience traits it helps most: self-awareness, self-regulation.
- Types that benefit most: all types, but for different reasons.

For moody warriors, it helps gain awareness of the mood cycles and what is happening internally when the mood is low, including any recurring body sensations, pain or discomfort. For wound-up warriors, it helps the awareness of the 'wound-up' state and those stress signatures. For exhausted warriors, it's being aware of the energy envelope before it is used up to avoid the boom–bust cycles of exhaustion from overdoing it. For scattered warriors, it helps in becoming more aware of the 'monkey mind' flitting between multiple things, making it hard to focus on any one of them.

This technique is also sometimes known as 'open monitoring meditation' when researchers try to classify it. Mindfulness meditation may also enhance 'mental error detection' too, which may help us see things more clearly and objectively. For example, if you are a moody warrior, you may tend towards 'glass half-empty' thinking or discounting the positives while amplifying the negatives. A daily few minutes of mindfulness can help you become aware of these 'thinking errors' and enhance multiple areas of resilience at once – such as mental and emotional resilience, help with social resilience/relationships and self-esteem.

Mindfulness has been shown to help conditions ranging from ADHD (which may affect scattered types more often) by helping to improve focus and mental function, to depression, helping with emotional stability in multiple studies.

If you suffer with chronic pain, regardless of your type, mindfulness has been shown to be a highly effective form of meditation to improve quality of life, pain and coping, especially since chronic pain starts to have a brain-amplification component involving the limbic or emotional brain which mindfulness helps to regulate.

MINDFULNESS SIMPLE PRACTICE INSTRUCTIONS

Find a comfortable place to sit, with your back supported if needed. Close your eyes and become aware of your breath, moving in and out of your body through the nose and down into the lungs and then up and out again through your mouth. Don't try to force or change your breathing or worry about the pattern. Just observe with curiosity what it does naturally. When thoughts come up, don't try to 'push them away' or 'blank your mind'. Instead, try to imagine your thoughts are like clouds passing by as you sit observing them from below without judging what is a good or bad thought. When you get distracted and notice it, simply say 'Oh well' and gently shift your attention back to your breathing again. Don't beat yourself up about getting sucked into a story or into your thoughts: it's natural. Every time you notice you're distracted and bring your attention back to the breathing, you have trained your brain towards a mindful state. Repeat this practice for a few minutes and then slowly bring your attention back into the room, feel your body sitting on the chair or floor and, taking one last deep breath with a long exhale, open your eyes again.

FAM (Focused Attention Meditation) focus/concentration Meditation

- Resilience traits it helps most: tolerance: when the brain is unable to filter out distractions, it can lose tolerance and become irritable.
- Types that benefit most: scattered warriors most of all, although helpful for all types.

This is often one of the first practices many meditators learn because it is easy to grasp quickly. This type of meditation involves choosing a core point of focus that can be the movement of your breath and its route in and out of the body, or a physical object to bring your attention back to when it drifts off. It can also involve focusing on a candle flame, a traditional Indian technique known as shatkarma or 'candle-gazing' meditation. This is one I was taught by my teacher and friend Peter Clifford, a yogic master who has studied in India for over fifty years and now teaches around the world. Another way of doing this type of practice is to choose a specific point on the wall to keep focusing back on when your attention drifts, or using a traditional mandala, a symbolic work of art often placed on a wall in a meditation room. Other meditation schools of thought incorporate this technique as one of the first lessons. For example, in vipassana, a form of silent meditation learned on retreat, focusing the attention strongly on the skin area just above the upper lip and below the nose – that's it – for a few days. This technique of focusing the attention is good for those who have trouble feeling overwhelmed or anxious with meditation from past experience, or who have tried mindfulness and found it very difficult to stick to long enough to see results. It may also work well for people who have trouble with focus and concentration as an initial skill to help focus the mind (if focus/attention was a challenge area for you!).

Loving Kindness/Compassion Meditation

- Resilience traits it helps most: empathy, self-regulation, self-esteem
- Types that benefit most: moody

Compassion and loving-kindness meditations have been shown to help improve mood and enhance empathy. The focus is on benevolent, loving or kind energy towards yourself and others. There are many compassion and loving-kindness meditation guides available online and in apps for free. Related practices are gratitude practices and forgiveness. All of these practices are especially helpful for a positive mood, positive sense of self and for those who suffer with depression. They help activate the left frontal lobe and specific brain regions associated with compassion and empathy.

COMPASSION/LOVING-KINDNESS SIMPLE PRACTICE INSTRUCTIONS

Start simply by sitting in a comfortable quiet spot and repeating the phrases 'May I be safe. May I be happy. May I be healthy. May I be free and live with ease.' You can experiment with similar statements that resonate with you, directed towards yourself first, then over time extending these feelings towards family members, then to friends and eventually even to strangers and those people you may dislike.

The Benson Technique and Mantra Meditation

- Resilience traits it helps most: self-regulation, flexibility
- Types that benefit most: wound-up warriors

This type of meditation involves including repeating a word or short phrase mentally over and over until the words lose their meaning. This method has been shown to improve anxiety and perceived stress. It has also been shown to induce an awake but relaxed, 'zenned-out' brain state involving more alpha-wave activity, something that wound-up warriors especially can benefit from. It can also lower blood pressure and enhance self-regulation. However, I have met many moody warriors who have faithfully practised a form of mantra meditation daily for many years and still had depression. In a review of multiple studies, depressed mood did not seem to shift with this type of meditation although it had other health benefits. So for moody warriors as a single practice, this is not my top choice.

One specific practice within this group is called TM, or Transcendental Meditation, and comes from a traditional vedic technique that is centuries old but was popularized by Maharishi Yogi in the 1950s in Rishikesh, India, where he famously taught the Beatles at his ashram and gave them each a secret personalized mantra to repeat while they meditated. The ashram is now derelict but still standing are some of the meditation huts which were used in its heyday. I had the chance to visit the ashram when I was in India on sabbatical years ago and filmed a video about it and a more 'generic' version of the technique which I have shared since with many of my patients.

A more generic version of this technique was adopted by Harvard researchers led by Dr Benson who investigated the relaxation response. He started out using a neutral word, 'one', and this had positive effects on his patients. However, he later discovered that a more emotionally associated word or phrase such as 'peace' or something even more specific to the meditator's specific spiritual or religious tradition (e.g. for someone of Christian faith, it could be 'Hail Mary', etc.) might work even better than using the word 'one' for everyone. As the phrase or word is repeated again and again in a single session, and also over a number of sessions as you log more hours of practice, the phrase can start to lose its conscious meaning to the brain after repetition. It's at this point that it goes from being quite similar to a focused attention meditation, where the brain is focused on the phrase itself, and takes on this more 'self-transcending' character as the words lose meaning.

BENSON TECHNIQUE SIMPLE PRACTICE INSTRUCTIONS

The Benson Technique involves choosing a specific short phrase that has some meaning to you if you have one based on your spiritual tradition, or a self-made mantra. You could also just use the word 'one' like Dr Benson first did with his patients or use something you create for yourself.

Once you have your word or phrase, you will repeat in your mind your word or phrase every time you exhale:

1. Focusing your attention on repeating the word or phrase on every exhale as you take relaxed belly breaths, sitting or lying in a comfortable position.
2. Adopting an attitude of patience and kindness to yourself when the mind wanders and just returning to repeating the word or phrase. It is normal for the mind to wander and does not mean you are 'doing it wrong'.

Body Relaxation Training

Resilience traits it helps most: self-regulation

There are other techniques that are more 'body focused', such as:

- PMR (progressive muscular relaxation): great for reducing body noise in wound-up warriors
- Rotation of awareness and body scans: good for all types but especially exhausted warriors.

These practices can be done lying down in a comfortable position using a guided recording until the practice becomes second nature, at which point many people find they no longer need an audio guide. These can be found easily for free online and in apps. A quick body-scan practice can be found in Part Three of this book under the mind–body week in the eight-week resilience quick-start programme.

Visualization: Getting to Know Your Best Self

- Resilience traits it helps most: self esteem, passion, flexibility, motivation.
- Types that benefit most: all types

There are many forms of visualization practices but one of my favourites is the 'best-self' practice. It's a practice that works well for every type because it is naturally about tailoring it to your individual needs. For example, if you are an exhausted warrior, part of the practice will likely be visualizing yourself energized in both body and mind. If you are scattered, you may visualize how organized and focused you are. Moody types will visualize experiences and habits that help cultivate more happiness, joy and passion, and wound-up warriors will picture themselves as calm and confident. This technique is a way to get acquainted with the more 'subconscious' aspects of yourself and also how you ideally see yourself in the future. You already possess the potential for all of the qualities in your future self, but just need to uncover them and remove any resilience roadblocks to start helping the best possible version of yourself to make more daily appearances. You can also think of it as your resilience visualization. It may feel silly at first, especially since visualizing ourselves in a positive future way isn't normally something we do as part of everyday life, and at first it can feel awkward or like you are not doing it right or are unable to focus or 'see anything'. Don't worry: it's normal. You will get better with a bit of practice and it will start to feel more natural because our brain's language is images, not words. This is a way that we can speak directly to our brain by speaking 'its language' in terms of visual images, sounds, smells and creating an emotive story for our brain to follow. The brain can respond to imagery that we create mentally in the same way as if it was really happening and light up the same brain areas. This is often used for professional athletes to help them perfect a physical skill with much less actual practice: they imagine themselves making that perfect putt or basketball freeshot or winning that race in the final few metres. This process of creating-your-best-self visualization also gives us important insider information about ourselves. It helps us become more aware of the interplay between our emotions, brain chemistry and even brainwave patterns and how they relate to our body sensations and any physical symptoms we may have. This process also helps us tap into our 'inner resource' or inner knowledge and can over time lead to having more 'Aha!' moments and help us resolve inner conflicts that we may have about ourselves and our self-image. These are a few important aspects of your resilience visualizations and how it works in the brain:

- Becoming completely absorbed in it: becoming very focused and absorbed in our visualization as we do it, so that we can create a rich 'story' of images, sounds, smells and even emotions
- Creating what is called an 'ideosensory experience' so that it seems real to the brain: the brain can respond to imagined sensory information just as well as the real thing. The classic example to practise with is imagining you have just picked a fresh lemon and how it tastes, smells and feels in your hand. Did your mouth start to water at the thought of the sour taste? Can you smell the citrusy notes even though it's not really there?
- Rehearsal: the more you envision something happening in your brain, the more powerful the message becomes. So, for example, if your future self eats a certain way or exercises every day or is fit and healthy, it sends a powerful repeat message to your brain that makes it more likely that you will stick with your resilience plan to make this future self a reality. It helps plant the 'mental seed' for change.

Visualization is not just for the hard-core meditators or sportspeople. Hundreds of studies have proven the benefits of visualization practices on almost all major physiological control systems in the body, from our heart and breathing rates to our metabolism, immune function, hormone levels including our stress-hormone cortisol, mood, pain levels and even sleep. In fact, of the nearly 2,000 studies on the influence of some form of visualization or imagery on health, 90 per cent showed a beneficial effect. The studies included benefits that are wide ranging: stroke recovery, PTSD, chronic pain, childbirth, cancer fatigue, quitting smoking, preparing for major surgery and anxiety. That rate of benefit is much higher than any single drug therapy we have to treat many of these same conditions. The best part is that visualization is a free skill we are all capable of, without any fancy training or skills.

By exploring what your best self looks like, you can understand what you really want out of life, what your best life looks like and what your top values are. This will help you know what to prioritize and know what are must-haves versus nice-to-haves when it comes to all aspects of your life. You can't do everything perfectly all the time, and in fact trying to do that is a recipe for burnout and actually lowering your resilience potential. For example, if you have a very busy work week, it may not be possible to cook from scratch every night and fit in getting to the gym or a yoga class too. If you are a busy parent with young children, it's probably not possible to meditate for an hour in peace and silence each day either.

When you go through this practice and you do meet your future self in your mind, what do they look like? How do they walk and carry themselves? What clothes are they wearing? Do they live in the city or in the countryside? What are their relationships like? What is their morning routine? How do they enjoy food? Do they have a particular job or occupation? How confident and happy are they? What are their passions or hobbies?

It was through doing this practice that I realized at the age of twenty-five that I wanted to start taking dance classes again as an adult, because it was actually a passion that I wasn't fully actualizing. So I gave up my gym membership and signed up to a dance studio instead. I still go twice a week and love it more than ever. Visualization offers you the chance to make your future self as rich in detail as possible, so you can get the deepest insight. This practice, if you have not done it before, may feel 'silly' or a bit too 'woo woo' for you. It may even feel a bit cringey to imagine your ideal self and life, or you might doubt you deserve it. Self-doubt and even a bit of 'impostor syndrome' can come up for many people when they do this practice. That's OK and totally normal, because intentional, positive introspection on this level isn't a part of daily life. However, I assure you this practice is backed by very credible science and not a waste of time. The good news is that the more you practise, the more those doubts will start to fade until they no longer intrude on your practice.

Visualization has been shown to improve performance under stress, improve mood and function in patients with fibromyalgia (a debilitating painful chronic condition) and has the ability to change health behaviours into more adaptive ones (i.e. more resilient ones!). Sports and task-specific visualization exercises can also enhance self-confidence and task performance in things from basketball free throws to surgical skill in doctors. You can repeat this practice as often as once a month (or more if you really enjoy it!) or as little as once a season to keep it current and keep your vision of your best self clear, reminding yourself that it is always there and accessible to you.

Obviously as you go through different life stages, your future self will likely change too. There are no rights or wrongs here. In fact, if an element of your future self starts to feel off, don't feel resistant to changing it. Maybe you thought you were a city person but after doing this practice a few times, you start to think you picture yourself living somewhere closer to nature, so go with it and see how it feels to experiment with this new version. The best part about visualization is that it can feel very real after our brain gets practised doing it, but it's a risk-free way to 'try on' something new – whether it's a new haircut, career, way of interacting with others, or any other aspect of your life where you want to gain more subconscious feedback about what might contribute to the best, most resilient and happiest version of you.

I advise doing this practice with a guided recording so you can fully relax your mind and become absorbed in the practice itself, at least for the first few times you do it until it starts to feel effortless. I still really enjoy listening to a recording version of this practice even though I have done it many times before.

FUTURE-SELF VISUALIZATION TIPS

Your future self doesn't have to be 'realistic' based on where you are right now. You don't need to worry about the details of how you will get there right now. This is your most ideal version of you, so go wild.

You may want to include some of these aspects in your visualization:

How you . . .
- Look
- Feel

- Interact with your family and friends
- Work life
- Daily routines
- Home environment
- How others see you
- Your emotions
- Accomplishments
- Health and vitality: what does that look and feel like for you?
- Ways you find fulfilment

The next step, now that you understand a bit about the how and why, is to set a time when you can try it out. Ideally, for the first time, try to leave twenty to thirty minutes if you can so that you have time to really focus and not rush the practice, which could last anywhere from five to twenty minutes (your call) followed by a few minutes of writing down some key points that you noticed afterwards in a paper journal or even in a notes app on your phone if you prefer an electronic record (less likely to get lost). After you feel comfortable with your visualization, you can repeat it as often as you wish, and only need to take five minutes for this practice. For example, on a Sunday you could set a reminder for the next four weeks to spend five minutes practising this visualization before bed. Some people find this practice very helpful and powerful and do a few-minutes version before drifting off to sleep each night, especially if they are working towards a specific goal over a set time frame. Nick and I have developed a little habit of doing our visualization practice together right before lights-out time in bed, as the last thing we think about before we drift off to sleep, for just two minutes. It is one of our daily rituals.

Yoga Nidra

- Resilience traits it helps most: self-regulation, self-awareness, flexibility, tolerance, empathy
- Types that benefit most: exhausted most of all, but all types can benefit

Yoga nidra is a mind–body practice known as an 'integrative' mind–body therapy. It has elements of mindfulness, body awareness, breath focus and visualization and sometimes loving kindness all rolled into one practice script. Yoga-nidra practices are usually done listening to a recording via headphones at home, at least when you are learning. Over time, you can run through the script mentally in your head without external guidance. However, I have found, doing the practice myself as well as recommending it to patients, that following a guided voice helps you sink deeper into the practice and get a feeling of deeper rejuvenation afterwards. Yoga nidra has a significant amount of research evidence to back up its efficacy, including helping to improve sleep, reduce stress, improve mood and self-esteem and enhance wellbeing.[2] It is a deeply rejuvenating practice and does not require a lot of mental energy since it does not require 'sharp' attention but simply an awake, relaxed, lying-down state while you listen to a recording. This is why I often recommend it to my patients who suffer with low-energy conditions such as chronic fatigue and fibromyalgia and why it is great for exhausted warriors.

My husband and I both learned this practice in India over a decade ago, where the teacher would do a live guided practice following the pranayama and asana training sessions. We both have very fond memories of a very hot, very basic ashram studio (sometimes on a concrete rooftop of a traditional house or ashram or, as was the case with one very senior swami we studied with, under a banyan tree outdoors with simple mats) where we were lying down listening to the swami guide the practice after a strenuous workout. Nick is also a trained clinical hypnotherapist and incorporates this practice into his hypnotherapy scripts. It also features in our personal practices at home where it is still one of our favourites, even though we have different resilience types. This was the practice Nick used to do for me, sometimes in a live version and he also made a recorded version for me to use when I was a stressed-out, sleep-deprived junior doctor to help me reset my sleep depth and cycles successfully after finishing a thirty-six-hour shift.

Moving Meditations

- Resilience traits it helps most: self-awareness, self-regulation, flexibility, tolerance
- Types that benefit most: all types, for different reasons. Wound-up warriors may find a movement practice that works on the fascia (connective tissue) and increases flexibility can help calm body noise. Exhausted types can use a very gentle form of movement to stay flexible and maintain fitness without exhausting themselves and going outside their energy envelope. Moody types can use it to 'activate' in the mornings, and scattered types can use the repetitive movements and coordination to focus their attention. Any exercise can become a mind–body practice when a mindful component is added.

Similarly, even a 'mindful' movement practice like going to a yoga class becomes less helpful if you spend the hour worrying that your downward dog doesn't look as pretty as someone else's! Becoming immersed in the activity is important to the meditative aspect. I get this from dance and some forms of yoga, and sometimes from running with a great playlist. Others find tai chi or a martial art, or even swimming, does it for them. However, there are also certain yoga poses and practices that may be best combined in a series for your type, based on the traditional uses for different poses and also based on the time of day and effect you want. For example, for wound-up and exhausted types, a restorative or yin yoga series done as part of the evening wind-down routine can work wonders for calming and restoring the nervous system. For moody and scattered types, starting the day with a short but energizing yoga series can work best to help set the tone for the day and get the mind and body ready to go.

One potential pitfall to be aware of is that the type of physical exercise or yoga style you may be initially drawn to may not be the most balancing for your type, especially when you get 'out of balance' when under more stress than normal. For example, wound-up warriors may be most drawn to a vigorous, fast-paced style of yoga such as ashtanga vinyasa, but may feel resistant to a more calming practice like yin, where you hold gentle poses for a long time. However, incorporating some yin sessions into a weekly routine instead of always going for 'max energy expenditure or calorie burn' can help balance and calm this type the most. To maximize your resilience, it is best to include a practice which buffers your challenges and helps you get out of ruts faster, whether that means doing some yin to help cultivate calm or alternately, if you are a moody warrior, doing an activating fast-paced vinyasa yoga or HIIT gym workout to help activate, which is what you need most, especially in the mornings.

IF EXERCISE COULD BE A PILL . . .

The reason physical movement and exercise, including everything from power walking to yoga and tai chi, is so good for us on so many levels is because it has a positive impact on our immune-system function, our brain chemicals that balance mood, focus and energy levels, and on our physical body and hormone systems – basically the immune–brain–inflammation matrix. If we could package exercise into a pill, it would be the miracle medicine everyone would be taking. Especially when it has a mind–body or meditative element. I tend to recommend types of exercise and movement that naturally have this mind–body component, like yoga, tai chi, dance or mindful walking. They all get the body moving but don't create too much strain on the system (which can increase stress hormone levels in some cases or deplete you further, especially if you are an exhausted warrior). My go-tos are simple hatha yoga routines that can be done at home for fifteen to twenty minutes a day and walking outdoors. Even if you hate gyms or working out, I have yet to meet someone who I haven't been able to help create a physical-movement practice that they enjoy doing and that fits gracefully into their lifestyle – even for the most exercise-averse!

'Meditative Movement' and Exercise Changes your Gene Expression

Moving mindful practices have unique effects on your gene expression or, in other words, what genes get turned on or off. Gene expression is the process of making proteins from your DNA building-block blueprint in your human genetic code. In fact, only 1 per cent of your genes in your genome (your DNA) get made into proteins. So that means that just because you have a gene for something, like a gene that predisposes you to diabetes or depression, it does not mean you are doomed to get that disease, as long as you are able to 'turn off' the negative genes so that they don't go on to making proteins that can make you ill. This modification of your gene expression is also known as 'epigenetics'. These modifications to the DNA are dynamic and, most importantly, reversible and related to both external and internal environmental influences. This epigenetic influence from physical exercise as well as meditation has been shown in multiple preliminary studies, including shutting off genes for everything from inflammation and cancer to neurodegenerative diseases.[3] Another recent study looked at a gentle lying-down yoga series for those suffering with chronic fatigue syndrome (CFS/ME) and discovered the practice changed their messenger RNA (biomarkers for CFS) after three months of daily twenty to thirty minute practice.[4] These are examples of why combining physical movement with a mind–body component is so powerful for resilience.

Somatic Intelligence and Resilience

Somatic, or 'body-intelligence'-based practices use simple body-focused practices designed to calm the mind and body under stress, using our breath, body movement and our five senses to bring us back into the present moment. These practices include breathwork (everything from a simple 'sigh' to release tension to actual breathing techniques to calm rather than energize), movement practices (such as dance, tai chi, or just free movement rolling around and playing on your living-room carpet!), and using touch (having a hug or receiving a relaxing massage). When I am feeling blocked mentally, trying to solve a problem or processing a difficult emotional experience, loss or change, one of my favourite self-care rituals is to go and have a dance followed by a massage. It completely resets my thinking and entire nervous system and never fails me. That is my personal 'somatic-reset' protocol. Other people may find dancing or getting a massage by a stranger even when they are a professional massage therapist invasive, annoying or stressful and prefer another method for decompressing using mindful movement.

Somatic intelligence is actually a form of intelligence just like we have emotional intelligence, and some of us are more naturally drawn towards somatic-intelligence body-based practices than others. Professionals like bodyworkers and osteopaths have a high amount of somatic intelligence, which is how they can often get great results with clients who may have tried many other therapies. The ones who are truly masters of these arts are very attuned to the subtle way of working with fascia, our body's layers of connective tissue, as well as the muscles and bones of the body. I go to an osteopath and an acupuncturist for 'tune-ups' myself periodically and more often when I have a niggle or when I was recovering from giving birth, for example. This type of therapy is something I also recommend to many of my patients who suffer with chronic pain but also conditions such as anxiety, stress, burnout and headaches as part of a holistic resilience plan.

It is also possible to hone your own somatic intelligence over time by doing mindful-movement practices like tai chi, yoga or dance, as well as mindful breathing practices. By tuning in to your body over time, you will be able to make subtle adjustments to your body position, posture and even breathing patterns and habits to relieve stress and tension, decrease anxiety and chronic pain and feel more physically and mentally resilient.

Yoga v. Other Forms of Mindful Movement and Exercise: What is Best?

One of the original purposes of yoga asana in India long before hot yoga was cool was to gain physical control over the body and regulate the nervous system against stress. And just like the four resilience types, traditionally your teacher would give you a practice just for you. Not everyone got the same thing: some were given practices that were more like ashtanga or vinyasa series, others more like yin and so on, depending on what each student needed to help balance their body and, even more importantly, their minds. This physical practice was also done to stretch the body and get it moving before sitting in meditation so people didn't become stiff. So the physical bit went hand in hand with the meditation.

Besides yoga, there are other physical practices that do the same thing, so don't sweat it if yoga doesn't do it for you. The common thread linking all of these practices is that each is a form of physical purposeful movement therapy, includes letting go of the conscious mind, and is non-exhaustive so it tones your nervous system back into balance instead of overwhelming it to exhaustion. This is what many people end up doing in the gym or extreme-fitness-type classes by over-exercising and pushing themselves to the extreme, which can ramp up the stress hormones, especially for certain types (exhausted and wound-up warriors in particular). You can do a home-based movement practised for ten to fifteen minutes three days a week and see a big difference over four to eight weeks or sooner. For mine, I do a combination of walking in nature and yoga/dance stretching exercises in the evening set to music.

THE FLYING GOOSE

This is one of my favourite short and simple, yet transformative, moving meditations which combines movement with breath. Any type can do it, but I especially love it for moody warriors to help 'wake up' the brain and body. It is best done in the mornings when you first wake to help activate the brain and body, or during the day after sitting for long periods of time at a desk to rejuvenate and get an energy burst without sugar or caffeine for those late-afternoon moments. It comes from the Indian five elements tradition and was taught to me by the yoga teacher I mentioned, Peter Clifford, who has specialized in this form of 'moving meditation' yoga for the past fifty years.

You start standing with feet shoulder distance apart and inhale as you bring the arms together over the head, keeping the legs straight, and stretch the arms upwards and bring them together. Then on the exhale, you bring the arms down through an arc movement while at the same time bending your legs down into a wide, deep-legged squat and as you come into the full squat at the end of the exhale, bring your arms crossed over each other in front of you. Then, you start to inhale, straighten the legs and bring the arms up the sides and back up above the head as you reach the top of your inhalation again. Repeat this movement

Cannabis and Psychedelic Yoga

For my medical cannabis patients suffering with complex chronic illnesses and, often, chronic pain and fatigue, any movement practice can be a huge challenge. But keeping the body moving as much as possible is so important for everyone. Often, to help connect to their bodies and make things feel more comfortable, using a small amount of vaporized cannabis before their practice, especially in the evening, can make a huge difference and make doing a bit of gentle yoga not only possible but also enjoyable. There are also those who use micro-dosing to enhance their yoga or physical mind–body practice experience (where legal). On my travels, I have also met wonderful yoga teachers who occasionally incorporate a low psychedelic dose of a substance into their practice to help them connect more deeply with themselves and their bodies and tune in to what their bodies really need most. At first I found this quite shocking when I first encountered it many years ago at a yoga retreat, but as I learned more about the medicinal uses of these substances it no longer seemed like a crazy idea, given the right (and of course legal) context. It's a fascinating use and as these substances become legal in more areas, I expect to see more 'cannabis yoga' and similar practices becoming increasingly openly discussed and possibly, eventually, even mainstream.

Meditation tips

HOW TO PRACTISE

You can keep your eyes open if you wish, but I usually advise trying to close your eyes if you are doing a sitting practice. Eyes closed appears better especially for less experienced meditators as it has been shown to be less distracting. The meditation position is another hotly debated topic: to sit or to lie down. Lying down is more relaxing so it may be better for wound-up and exhausted warriors. Sitting may work best for moody and scattered types, since sitting upright helps maintain focus and upright body posture may confer subconscious positive messages about our self-construct to the brain. Especially if you are an exhausted warrior and choose to lie down, and fall asleep when you are practising, don't worry. Even if you get a few minutes of practice in and then a short power nap, this is restorative and beneficial. As your energy gets better, you will find you will be able to maintain alertness longer and longer without forcing it.

WHEN TO PRACTISE

You can choose to do it either as part of your morning routine, at lunchtime or before bed, depending on what suits your lifestyle and schedule the best. I prefer to do mine in the evening as part of my post-screen-shut-off wind-down routine before bed, or sometimes at lunchtime to help reset for the afternoon. My husband, however, prefers to do his in the morning. This isn't surprising since my main resilience type is wound-up warrior and his is scattered. I have found that choosing a morning practice time works best for many scattered and moody warrior types. Wound-up warriors do best as part of the pre-bed routine. Exhausted warriors often have to find the time of day where they feel like they have the most energy. That could be as soon as they wake up, mid-morning or lunchtime for others.

Formal v. Informal Practice

The five-to-ten-minute practice you do each day, ideally at the same time, is called your 'formal' mind–body practice, meaning it is a time you set aside to focus only on that and nothing else. Research as well as my own personal experience with meditation and over a decade of clinical experience using mind–body practices with patients has shown that we have to keep up our practice to keep reaping the brain and resilience benefits. Otherwise the brain and mind can slowly 'slip' back into old, less resilient habits again, which make us more susceptible to stress. However, the more months and years you practice, the more entrenched the positive brain changes will be and you may find yourself automatically doing some aspects of the practice throughout your day, as they become 'second nature'. This is your 'informal' practice, meaning your brain will automatically launch into some of the positive techniques or 'programmes' as you go about your day. For example, if you do a formal gratitude practice each day called 'Three Good Things' where you mentally rehearse or even write down (bonus points!) three good things that happened that day or that you are grateful for, your brain will start thinking of more even outside your ten-minute window. That's because that is what our brains do: they try to be helpful. And if you are in a more positive, grateful mood, the brain will try its best to find more 'concordant' thoughts and emotions to match your mood – i.e. more positive, grateful pearls. The same is true if you are a wound-up warrior and you start regularly practising the relaxation response meditation. You then feel less anxious and calmer and the brain wants to make that feeling last. This means that your brain will automatically shift into a more mindful, relaxed and resilient state when faced with daily stressors instead of reflexively reacting negatively by tensing up, making the breathing more shallow and going into fight-or-flight mode like you used to.

Combining Techniques Together

Traditionally, before we had modern researchers that have taken a specific technique and made it 'mainstream', such as Jon Kabat-Zinn did with mindfulness, individual meditation or mind–body techniques were not taught in isolation. They were instead part of a bigger framework and deep tradition, such as in the many different schools of Buddhist meditation. In these traditional systems, the techniques were taught over many years in a specific order and then combined with other practices as students built up their skill level. To reap the resilience and health benefits of a mind–body practice, however, it is not necessary to spend hours a day, or even one hour a day. With our own practice, my husband Nick and I often combine a few specific techniques into a single short practice, with a recording Nick has made so we can listen to it easily. This is a way of deepening a practice, should you have the time or inclination, like a mini modern version of the traditional way of doing things without needing hours a day and with the goal of resilience in mind. However, even just one very simple practice done for a few minutes each day can make huge changes happen in as little as just under two months (eight weeks).

If you already have a practice you like but it is different from the one suggested for your type, you can keep your current one and add a few minutes of a second technique to expand your practice further and create one of these combination or integrated practices tailored just for you. There is no right or wrong way to use these practices, or a same way that works for everyone.

How Long Does it Take Before I Feel Different?

There are some techniques which may be most important for your resilience type, but regardless of the one you choose, you do need to keep at it to see changes. I recommend for the first eight weeks committing to ten minutes each day to train the brain in these new 'brain skills'. In most studies on meditation and mind–body practices, brain changes were seen in eight weeks of daily practice of between six and twenty minutes a day, with longer sessions being slightly more effective or leading to more changes in some studies. After eight weeks, your practice will settle but it is important to keep it going most days if possible to maintain the benefits, although some people may be able to condense it down further. Many people find they really start to enjoy those set-aside minutes as they gain more expertise and can get into their 'flow' state by doing their practice, and that it makes them feel quite powerful, knowing they have this ability to self-regulate no matter what stresses life throws at them. It makes it easier to deal with the uncertainties of life. Some people will also find they benefit from longer sessions, and you can always expand the practice on days when you have more time, but don't stress if you can't. The key is being consistent with your practice and it is better to do five minutes most days than spend a whole hour just once a week.

PARADOXICAL ANXIETY REACTIONS TO BREATHWORK AND MIND–BODY PRACTICES

I have had patients in my practice over the years who cannot tolerate many forms of meditation, at least when they are beginners. For them, it can trigger a panic attack or less severe feelings of anxiety, discomfort and feeling mentally and emotionally 'unsafe'. It is sometimes also called paradoxical anxiety, meaning anxiety when you think you should feel the opposite – relaxed – particularly if you are a wound-up warrior. A possible explanation for why this happens is that our breathing muscle, the diaphragm, is getting used in a new way when we do deep breathing for the first time. The diaphragm is connected to our nervous system directly and the practice can stress it temporarily until the nervous system adjusts. Another possible explanation is that bringing your attention to your breathing, which may have been quite shallow and tense for many years, brings more conscious awareness to this stress tension and sense of breath shallowness, which can bring up more feelings of anxiety temporarily.

If this happens, take a break and then try the practice a few hours later but for a shorter time. So if you started with one minute, reduce it to thirty seconds until this length of time starts to feel comfortable. Other forms of mind–body practices may also cause a temporary but uncomfortable feeling of anxiety as the brain adjusts in some people. Again, just back off and restart the practice you have chosen for a shorter amount of time the next day and as it begins to feel more comfortable, you can build up your time again. On the other hand, if you are a moody or exhausted warrior, you may notice that certain breathing practices actually make you feel more energized or revitalized, even in the first days you practise. Scattered warriors are the least likely to have these anxiety reactions. Their biggest challenge is sitting still and being patient as they learn these new brain skills without rushing.

Breathwork

How We Breathe

The way we breathe controls so much more than getting oxygen into our lungs. How we breathe affects our nervous-system balance. Poor breathing patterns can contribute to issues for each resilience type: it can bring on anxiety, lower energy levels, make us feel sluggish or low and affect mental clarity. Something as simple as what is called 2:1 breathing, which means bringing a gentle focus on making your exhale twice as long as your inhale, has a calming and stabilizing effect on the nervous system for all types. Many of us reverse this ratio during the work day, sitting at our desk with stress building up, lengthening our inhales instead, which creates even more stress in the nervous system. Another common breathing 'error' is sucking in the belly on the inhale, or trying to suck in our bellies constantly, which can prevent our breathing muscle from moving as it should and cause issues ranging from anxiety, or even panic, to pain in the back.

Breathwork is the use of different ways of breathing, from the sound of the breath to the length of an inhale and exhale and the use of our breathing muscle, the diaphragm, as an entire class of mind—body practices. I could devote an entire book to just breathing alone. I have years of experience with many, if not most, of these techniques and have studied with different breathwork teachers all over the world on my resilience-medicine journeying.

Any of these breathing techniques can also be used as your one-minute resilience-reset practice. My two favourite resets are the healing breath (when I'm feeling stressed or anxious) and kapal-bhati (when I need some energy). I come back to them again and again and they always help me feel better almost instantly. Patients to whom I have recommended these breathing practices to help with conditions ranging from anxiety and burnout to depression and chronic pain management over the years have found the same.

They are incredible medicine and an almost instant window to our mind–body connection, a reminder of how powerful a single minute's practice can be to shift our resilience potential, no matter how big the current challenges.

Why do breathwork practices work so well across so many different health issues? It has to do with helping tone our autonomic nervous system (ANS) balance by stimulating and moving our breathing muscle, the diaphragm. The diaphragm has a special nerve running through it called the vagus nerve that is critical in maintaining that ANS balance between the sympathetic nervous system and the parasympathetic, just like we learned about in Part One. When we don't use our diaphragm properly, it can upset this balance. On the other hand, intentional breathing practices, called pranayamas in the Indian tradition, can help the diaphragm move as it should again, even when we are not actively practising the technique. It can also help shift our nervous system out of fight-or-flight, especially using the calming techniques listed, in under a minute. Sometimes, my patients combine things like vaporized low THC or CBD hemp cannabis flower before they do their practice to help enhance the effects they feel, especially for wound-up warriors to help calm anxiety fast.

Some pranayamas can be learned easily in a few minutes at home by just following the written instructions (e.g. the healing breath, bee breath, nadi shodhana). Others are best learned with a teacher and/or videos to follow that demonstrate and fully explain the technique. This is especially true if you are not familiar with deep diaphragmatic breathing techniques. Many yoga teachers are trained in some of these and can offer assistance to get you started, so then you can keep practising at home too. Holotropic breathing and similar rebreathing sessions (sometimes called 'rebirthing' breathing) are generally done under guidance from a skilled practitioner, either in a group or one-to-one.

The Healing Breath

This is a calming breath where you inhale slowly and deeply while expanding the belly, inhaling through the nose, and then exhaling slowly through the mouth while making a gentle *haaaaaa* sound on the exhale. Try to make the exhale longer than your inhale, but do not force it. If you start to feel short of breath, do the practice more gently and stick to the exhale length that feels most comfortable for you.

Bee Breath

Also known as bhramari. This breath restricts the senses of sight and hearing and creates a sense of calm that can help reduce feelings of overwhelm.

Use your thumbs to close the ears and the first two fingers to cover the eyes. Keeping the mouth closed, take a deep breath in. Then exhale with a sound of *hmmmm* or *auumm*, which should create a significant buzzing or vibration effect, especially with your ears and eyes closed.

Nadi Shodhana

Also known as alternate-nostril breathing, this is a yogic breathing practice used for thousands of years in the yoga tradition to 'balance' the nervous system. Traditionally it was taught that regular dedicated practice over months can help bring better inner balance. Even one session can lead to feelings of calm clarity.

Essentially it is done by closing one nostril at a time and breathing through each one alternately. Like many practices, having a teacher show you in person or watching a video the first time can be much easier than written instructions (which make it sound overly complicated; it is quite simple in practice). Traditionally the exact hand placements involve two fingers on the forehead in between the eyebrows to rest while the other fingers on the same hand rest on the side of the nose to open and close the nostril, and then changing, but an easier version is just using the thumb to block and unblock one nostril at a time as follows:

Sit in a comfortable position, inhale gently and exhale all the air out.

As you exhale, use your right thumb to close your right nostril.

Then inhale through your open left nostril and then close it at the top of your inhale with your fingers.

Open the right nostril and exhale through this side (e.g. exhale through the right nostril).

Then close the right nostril again and repeat.

This is one cycle.

Ujjayi Breath

Most often associated with ashtanga or vinyasa styles of yoga, but the breath can be done on its own too. It involves partially constricting the throat so you make a subtle ocean or rushing sound while practising deep diaphragmatic breathing.

Kapalbhati

Also known as cleansing breath, where the exhale forcefully uses the diaphragm strength to exhale and then let the inhale happen passively. This technique is often taught in kundalini yoga. Focus on the exhalation using the diaphragm and the inhale will happen naturally without needing to force it. Avoid generally if you are pregnant, or have certain health conditions (e.g. heart issues).

This is the practice I did every day for five months when my husband Nick and I spent nearly half a year living in rural India, studying with traditional teachers. When I got back to Vancouver, everyone kept asking if I had had botox or 'done something' because I looked so 'calm and radiant'! I kept up the practice every day for nearly a year after that and although I don't do it every day any more, it is my go-to for an energy pick-me-up during the work day. Those who should avoid this practice generally include those with high blood pressure, heart issues, stroke, certain eye conditions (detached retina), hernias or pregnancy.

Bhastrika

Also known as the 'bellows breath', where both the inhale and exhale are somewhat forceful, using the diaphragm to push air in and out, giving the breathing muscle a workout. You begin in a comfortable seated position. Then take a deep breath in, and breathe out forcefully, using the diaphragm. Immediately after the exhale, breathe in with the same force. Inhale and exhale repeatedly, using the diaphragmatic muscles. Those who should avoid this practice again generally include those with high blood pressure, heart issues, stroke, certain eye conditions (detached retina), hernias or pregnancy.

Holotropic Breathwork

Originally developed by psychiatrists Stanislav and Christina Grof in the 1970s to achieve altered states of consciousness without using psychoactive substances for therapeutic and wellbeing purposes. Drs Grof also studied the therapeutic uses of LSD (see the chapter on power plants for more info on this, page 159) but wished to explore an alternative to achieving similar 'psychedelic' healing states using non-drug approaches as studying LSD became more restricted. It involves deep controlled breathing without a pause at the top of inhaling or after exhaling, and involves voluntary 'hyperventilation'. It is generally safe for most healthy people but should be avoided if pregnant or if you have a medical condition (to be safe, check with your doctor first). It should be done, at least initially, with a trained guide. Participants report it being helpful for healing and personal growth and can have profound personal insights and improvements in symptoms like anxiety and low mood. There have been a few published case reports of successful medical use as a treatment in severe treatment-resistant depression and with those suffering from addiction.

High-tech Mind–body Techniques

In addition to traditional 'low-tech' meditation and mind–body techniques, recent advances in neuroscience have led to 'high-tech' brainwave and biofeedback-assisted mind–body training techniques. We found that people who had difficulty meditating before responded very well to neurofeedback, which uses visual and audio feedback on what your brain is doing in 'real time' to help reach a more balanced state and can be tailored to the person and the issue. For example, for wound-up warriors, there are calming protocols that work on reducing dysfunctional 'hi-beta' activity in certain areas of the brain. For those suffering with low mood, a protocol to 'wake up' the left frontal lobe can be very helpful. For those with chronic fatigue, burnout and exhaustion there is a 'deep-state' restorative protocol that helps the brain access a deep, healing meditative state in between sleep and waking called the 'alpha-theta crossover state'. The downside was that the technology that accurately reads these brainwaves and delivers training is very expensive and difficult to use, unlike the consumer versions available at a much lower price (just under a thousand pounds) that unfortunately are not quite accurate enough (yet). You also need many sessions to get a sustained result, just like regular meditating, since the equipment is simply training the brain to learn how to access the more adaptive states. It doesn't put 'anything into' the brain or 'zap' the brain. The expense and difficulty in delivering the service was the major drawback in the end. My husband and I both still use our equipment at home occasionally to help with energy and improve coordination for dance (me) and help with focus (Nick).

Another 'high-tech' tool we used at our wellness centre was something called HRV or heart rate variability training. This is a much cheaper technology than the brain neurofeedback. It consists of a small earclip connected to a handheld device which measures the pattern of heartbeats over time. There is some research to show that resilience heartbeat patterns are different from those in patients suffering from low resilience states, severe stress, anxiety and depression, and these can be picked up using this biofeedback device. The idea is that, using breathing and feedback about your heartbeat patterns, you can learn to influence this pattern in a positive, more resilient direction over time. We found using it with clients that it works better for some people than others, but it is an affordable technology that can be used at home as a meditation and relaxation tool. Another similar tool is called a cranial electrotherapy stimulation device (CES), which is more expensive than HRV devices but still under £500 and can be helpful especially for wound-up warriors but also for any type for calming anxiety, helping with mood and getting to sleep, and has published evidence for its positive effects.

These are three additional tools you may wish to consider on your resilience journey.

Mental Exercises for Cultivating Resilient Thoughts and Emotions Based on Your Type

Mental resilience is all about creating ways of thinking and doing that can help boost your ability to navigate life's more challenging times and happenings with less stress. It is not the same as 'mental toughness' or how hard you can push yourself. It's not about beating yourself up about not doing enough or being perfect. It's more about creating mental and emotional flexibility to help us bounce back from life's many speed bumps. Depending on your type, there are different mental exercises that may be most helpful for you to retrain unhelpful thinking patterns or mental habits we all fall into to some degree.

These exercises all have a large body of research behind them and are a combination of practices from positive psychology and cognitive behavioural therapy or CBT, and all help cultivate at least one, often several, of the top-ten resilience temperament traits from Part One. Choosing just one of these and putting them into practice for a minute each day can help your brain pick up a new more adaptive mental habit to replace a less resilient one over time. Working with a CBT therapist or positive psychologist to really put these into action can also help too, but many of these mental tools can be used as part of self-care and are also available in mental wellbeing apps too.

I have included these in the mind–body chapter because although they are slightly different from meditating, they are mind–body interventions that can help create more resilient thinking and emotional responses with practice. They work in slightly different ways from most meditation techniques, but mindfulness has many similarities and many of these exercises work well with mindfulness too.

In other cases – if you are a wound-up warrior, for example – you may use a calming meditation technique like the Benson Technique or the healing breath first to help reduce stress and anxiety in the moment and then once you are feeling calmer, try one of these more 'cognitive' strategies to help reduce worry or catastrophizing, so that when you encounter a similar stressor or situation in the future, your brain can respond differently and doesn't get so wound up. They can then work together as different brain 'thinking' skills alongside the mind–body practices we have explored so far in this chapter.

Wound-up Warriors

Identify catastrophic thinking and 'decatastrophize'. Wound-up warriors tend to think about the worst-case scenario and get worked up and stressed and worry about it more than any other type. Identifying when this happens is the first step, and then creating the opposite to this catastrophic ending in your mind and reminding yourself that the worst-case scenarios rarely happen.

Identify 'thinking errors' about worrying. Many wound-up warriors believe on some level, often a subconscious one until they really bring it into more conscious awareness, that worrying actually helps change outcomes or can make things work out better. This false belief that worrying about something actually makes things better or can change what happens makes people become attached to their worrying habit. Try telling yourself that you can safely let go of worrying or mentally put it in your 'worry box' and place it to the side in your mind. You can also try thanking you brain for alerting you to this worry for its attempt to be helpful, but remind yourself you actually don't need to worry about that thing right now and don't need to hold on to that worry any longer: you've logged it and assessed it as a non-issue. It is safe to let that worry go now.

Visualize coping well in a stressful situation. Wound-up warriors tend to worry about their ability to cope with stress and doubt their ability to tolerate stress. This technique to enhance your self-belief in your coping ability is sometimes called 'exposure visualization'. You picture the event or situation that was creating worry or stress and visualize yourself doing a great job (if it's worry about a work presentation) or having a great time (if it's going to a party where you don't know many people). Try to make the visualization as rich as possible – see the best-self visualization section (page 199) for more tips.

Check the people-pleasing. Wound-up warriors as well as exhausted warriors both tend to be overly tuned in to other people's needs and emotions. Empathy is good, but focusing mainly on other people's needs and constantly seeking approval can lead to anxiety and difficulty relaxing and winding down and also to exhaustion. If this sounds familiar, try asking yourself:

* Am I looking after my own needs and putting myself first? If not, am I going to extreme lengths to please someone else at the cost of my own wellbeing?

Exhausted Warriors

USE ENERGY ENVELOPES

Energy envelopes or the energy 'check-in' can help you see how charged-up your batteries feel in terms of both mental and physical energy. This was used originally to help patients who suffer with chronic fatigue syndrome or ME to reduce energy crashes and can take a few different forms. One of my close friends and colleagues, Dr Elena Miller, took this concept of the energy envelope one step further to help herself recover her energy levels after battling and surviving stage-four cancer twice. You assign even simple low-stimulation activities such as watching TV a point value. More points equal more energy needed. Once she'd used up her total number of points each day, she would then try to absolutely minimize her energy output for the rest of that day. The only thing that had zero points was actually sleeping. As she slowly regained her strength, she allowed herself a few more points (i.e. expanded her energy tank) each day. When she had an energy crash or setback, she would then go back to having fewer points per day again.

I used a similar system to help recover my energy after I had severe dengue fever a second time while in Bali. Even things like talking on the phone to friends and family, eating a meal and reading had an energy output, so even these activities were 'rationed'. It took weeks for me to fully recover, and each week I added on higher-point activities and expanded my envelope bit by bit.

SET FIRM BOUNDARIES

Exhausted warriors may also have trouble setting boundaries and this can zap energy levels. When you start to prioritize your own needs and set boundaries, you will actually end up feeling less drained and have less 'compassion' fatigue. This means you will actually have a greater capacity to do nice things and think of others too, from a place of security and confidence rather than feeling constantly obligated, which causes fatigue.

Practise saying no more. If you tend to have limited energy reserves, the more you take on, the more energy you use up and you can easily end up overextended. It can feel really uncomfortable or even selfish to say no. However, far from being selfish it is part of taking care of your energy tank. Check in with yourself and your 'bandwidth' before saying yes to something, whether it's an extra project at work or a commitment to a loved one or friend. Take a deep breath or a resilience reset using the healing breath and then ask yourself if you are taking on too much by saying yes. Say no nicely but firmly instead, without an apology or overexplaining.

Moody Warriors

AVOID ISOLATION

Moody warriors may tend to isolate themselves when under stress more than other types, as a coping mechanism. Breaking the cycle of isolation by calling a friend or spending more time with family or a furry friend can help to decrease stress and enhance your social connectivity, one of the top-ten resilience traits too over time.

Work on your 'learned optimism'. In Part One we learned about the top resilience temperament trait of optimism, where moody types may struggle most. Our brains tend to have a built-in negativity bias which means we may pay more attention to the negative, and moody types may feel this more strongly than other types. It is, however, all shiftable. When moody types are in balance, they are also the life of the party and highly sociable, so overcoming this negativity bias can help bring out their best qualities with a few simple practices.

OPENING AND CLOSING DOORS METHOD

To cope with changes with more optimism, the first step is to acknowledge the hard emotions, the pain and loss, so that stuff doesn't get pushed down and repressed. After that, mentally reframing the change can shift the focus to the positive. This process can take less than five minutes, it doesn't have to be a novel!

Instructions: write down in a journal or smartphone, or review mentally, these steps:

A door that just closed for me/recent change/loss was . . .

This made me feel . . . (sad, worried, dejected, grief, pain, etc.)

A new door that could open could be . . .

The possibility of this new door opening makes me feel . . . (hopeful, happy, satisfied, motivated, etc.)

THREE GOOD THINGS AND THE GRATEFUL JAR METHODS

The next practice is all about gratitude and noticing the positive to shake up that moody-warrior negativity bias. It's also something that is helpful for those who struggle with positive mood balance. In the first practice, Three Good Things, you end each day with a one- or two-minute practice to acknowledge out loud (and bonus points for jotting it down in a journal!) three good things that happened that day. They can be anything from being able to enjoy your morning cup of coffee to having a call with a friend, to even something small like saying hello and receiving a smile in return from a stranger on the tube on your morning commute. In the Grateful Jar version, you write on little scraps of paper one to three things you are grateful for each day and pop it in the jar. When you go through a challenging time, you can pull out the jar, which fills up over time and read them over to get that feel-good vibe going in the brain again and break the negativity loop.

Scattered Warriors

Scattered warriors are creative visionaries but frustratingly they often have problems seeing their great ideas and plans through to fruition. However, this type's superpower for creative problem-solving can shine when the ability to focus and keep mental clarity is honed with some simple 'brainhacks'.

BREAKING THINGS DOWN

Scattered types tend to get overwhelmed by big projects since they tend to see the big picture and are generally quite creative, both positive attributes but sometimes these traits come at the expense of being able to break things down into bite-sized, manageable pieces and chunks of work.

RECOGNIZE FAULTY BELIEFS ABOUT SIGNS YOU SHOULD QUIT

Scattered warriors more than other types may have the emotional feeling or belief that experiencing feelings of frustration or confusion are signs that they should quit what they are doing. This leads to not finishing things. Instead, when you identify these feelings, remind yourself that these are signs you are learning and a positive sign as well as a normal part of the learning process and the road to mastery.

CLARIFYING AND VISUALIZING GOALS

Especially for scattered warriors, goal-setting is really important for staying on track mentally and staying clear about what is really important to you. This can be done very formally and take an entire afternoon, or it can be done in just a few minutes by asking yourself what your top three goals are for this week, and maybe the top goal for today. It could be anything from finishing a work project milestone to cooking a loved one dinner or doing the laundry, but make sure it's something you can do and then tick off to give yourself that hit of dopamine or satisfaction brain chemicals scattered types need a lot of to stay motivated and clear.

CREATE HYPERFOCUS OPPORTUNITY WINDOWS IN YOUR DAY

You may find that you have the ability to 'hyperfocus' when you are really interested in something, like many people of this type. So creating windows of hyperfocus in the work day for a task or project you are excited about, to utilize this strength, can maintain momentum and reduce boredom. Many scattered types find that they work well in these 'bursts' whereas other types may do better working at the same, slower but very steady pace.

Mind–body Passion Practices: Why Everyone Needs A 'Fun Prescription' Too

As we learned in Part One, passionate 'zest' is one of the top resilience traits for all types. This relates to bringing more joy, fun and passion back into daily life. It doesn't mean needing to 'go wild' or become a hedonist, but is more about creating daily and weekly moments and activities that meet this human need.

How Modern Medicine Forgot About Joy and Passion

Incorporating fun and passionate zest into health is something that my profession of medicine kind of forgets about a lot of the time. It's one reason why many docs are not so great at helping their patients break out of the ruts we all get into from time to time, when we can start to feel like life is just 'meh'. It's not your doctor's fault. It's just not part of medical culture or training to talk about what were thought of as 'fluffy' things like passion and purpose, being emotionally connected or making 'heart and head' decisions unless you are a psychotherapist. It feels uncomfortable or even unprofessional to many doctors to discuss these things. However, the best doctors I know are the ones who manage to connect on this level with their patients in addition to being really good at analysing facts and test results. Their patients feel empowered and have a better quality of life when faced with chronic illnesses.

No matter what your type, it is equally important to inject a bit of fun into daily life. Fun is another form of mind–body practice because of the profound effects joy and passion have on our resilience. Children are naturally good at this. For them, learning is play. But for adults, we often stop prioritizing these softer skill sets because life gets busy and the responsibilities of adulthood make it harder to fit everything in. When I ask my patients what they do for fun and are passionate about besides work, they often reply 'I'm too busy' to worry about that. Some people may also feel guilty (hello, wound-up warriors!) for taking time for things that society may deem 'frivolous' or 'unessential'. But joy and passion are absolutely essential ingredients for brain resilience. Introducing an element of playfulness back into life can also help boost creativity, increase our sense of freedom rather than 'feeling trapped' in life and help the brain shake up stress and worry loops. This is why practices such as laughter 'yoga' have taken off in recent years in the west amongst respectable adults. Get your natural 'feel-good' hormones going by playing! Do cartwheels, draw a picture, sing, dance, let yourself be silly with friends, whatever it means to you to play.

Cultivating more passion and fun in your life can look slightly different based on your type. For example, wound-up warriors can begin to feel less connected to their passion and purpose if they let stress levels get out of control and feel constantly 'wound up'. That is because the stressed, 'jacked-up' brain state can shut down brain circuits related to creativity, joy and passion. For moody warriors, joy and passion are particularly important in breaking low-mood ruts, so actively choosing and scheduling (even though it sounds counter-intuitive) an activity you used to enjoy but somehow stopped doing, whether it's playing a musical instrument or seeing friends each week for coffee, is crucial to wake up your brain to joy again. Even if you don't feel like doing it, you will nearly always feel better when you do. If you are an exhausted warrior, you may have a different challenge in that some of your favourite activities in the past may be too energy-zapping currently. So instead of crossfit you may want to explore with curiosity a new hobby that is less energy-demanding.

It could be anything from photography to enjoying music in some way. For scattered types, it's about choosing a creative outlet, since being creative is often a superpower, and then scheduling it in so it happens regularly.

Getting More 'Aha!' Moments

One of the things I started to experience myself and my patients all report back to me is that they have more 'Aha!' moments' when they start reconnecting to their passions. 'Aha!' moments are moments and periods of dramatically enhanced mental clarity, calm focus and creative innovation. I have had some of my best 'Aha!' moments after I do my dance practice.

These are some passion activities you can use to trigger 'Aha!' moments in the brain based on the latest research from Dr Herbert Benson and Dr Sarah Lazar at Harvard University:

- Dancing or 'free movement' to music at home
- Gardening
- Drawing/sketching/painting
- Singing/chanting
- Listening to music
- Watching a play/concert/dance performance/theatre show that you find emotionally 'moving' for you
- Going to see an art installation, gallery or exhibit
- Getting away for a weekend and putting yourself in a novel environment to break your physical and mental routines
- Walking in nature

How to do it:

1. Write down your favourite things to do, hobbies or even games that you loved when you were a child or adolescent.
2. Brainstorm how you can bring aspects of those interests or activities into your life again and schedule a 'fun' appointment into the calendar each week for thirty minutes minimum.

Mind–body practices need not be complicated. They can be simple, practical things we can do to make us feel a bit happier, less stressed and more resilient in hectic modern life. They are also accessible to everyone once you know where to start. When you tap into your built-in but often forgotten-about relaxation response for just a few minutes each day, great things happen.

PART 3

TAKING ACTION

CHAPTER 8

THE EIGHT-WEEK RESILIENCE PROGRAMME

So now you know all about your resilience type and are armed with the most powerful toolkit to help you become the most resilient version of yourself. Becoming more resilient won't happen overnight, so be gentle. The only rule is to be kind and compassionate to yourself as you embark on your resilience journey. If you do just that, you have already taken a huge step towards creating more resilience for yourself.

I've included this programme in the book for those who may feel they want a bit of week-by-week guidance on putting all the things they've learned into action. I understand that making these changes can feel overwhelming, and this is simply a way to help make it seem a little easier. This is by no means the only way to use the recommendations in the book, so please don't feel like you need to commit to the intensity of such a programme to reap any benefits. The programme is simply a tool for you to use if it's helpful.

When I work with my patients and clients, I introduce them to their resilience plan step by step and we generally make a few changes at a time to avoid causing more stress and overwhelm. This is especially important for exhausted warriors, who are most prone to taking on too much for their current 'energy envelope'.

Eight weeks is my suggested time frame for the resilience programme, but you can stretch it out and take more time for each stage. For example, if you are extremely busy you may need to do things less intensely. That's fine, you can repeat a particular week for multiple weeks, a month or even longer if you need to. This is especially true for the weeks that involve interventions such as diet change and, especially, mind–body practice, since these take time and considerable effort, especially at the start, until they become a habit. Other changes like adding a supplement, CBD or cannabinoid are simpler because they are something you simply need to 'take' each day, not block time to actually 'do', such as adapting meals to fit a new way of eating or starting to meditate. For example, for your mind–body practice, the optimal amount of time based on the research is around twenty minutes a day especially in the initial learning phase of the first two to eight weeks. This really helps your brain 'lock in the learning'. But many people can only fit in five minutes a day and that's totally OK too. The practices and benefits will just take longer to sink in, so just be a bit more patient with the results.

Also keep in mind that often less is more when it comes to 'doing' things. It can be a good idea to feel you have mastered each week (or phase if you are taking longer than a week) before moving on to the next one, to avoid overwhelm or create *more* stress by overscheduling and piling on 'more things' when you are still in the learning phase of the last one. Each week (or phase) builds on the progress from the previous one, so we stack our resilience hacks up as we go along over the next eight or more weeks.

With these things in mind, let's outline a typical eight-week plan.

A WOMEN'S HEALTH NOTE

As you go through the next eight weeks, it is likely that this will be nearly two menstrual cycles if your cycle lengths are around twenty-eight days. As you go through the different phases of your cycle, you may want to notice any changes in how you feel at different times of the month. It is normal and natural for every type to experience cyclical changes in things like energy, feeling stressed versus calm, mental clarity and mood. This may affect things like your food cravings, energy you have for physical movement and exercise, how easy it is for you to do your meditation practice and the dose of things you may want to 'take', like CBD, adaptogens and even magnesium. For example, women who experience PMS may find that increasing things like CBD and calming adaptogens like ashwagandha the week before your period may help ease symptoms. Or that extra magnesium and calcium can help if you have bad period cramps. (See the supplements and botanicals chapter, page 141, as well as the cannabinoids chapter, page 159, for details on women's health supplements.)

Week 1: Circadian Rhythm Reset and Supplements

We will start by focusing on sleep and resetting your sleep/wake cycle to the optimal rhythm. Sleep is one of the bedrocks of resilience since it is so critical to making our brain, immune system and body work properly. It is very difficult to thrive without good sleep. This process is important for all types but especially for wound-up and exhausted warriors, who tend to have the highest sleep support needs.

The other thing we will start this week, if applicable to you, is resilience supplements. I like to start out with supplements too because it's something easy you can do to get a quick win in terms of resilience, especially when you tailor them to your type. Some supplements take weeks to take effect, so the sooner you try them, the sooner you will know if they are helping and it's something that doesn't take a lot of time in the day or loads of effort. The downside is that they have a monetary cost, so if you are on a budget, you can hold off on them for now and just focus on the core sleep reset.

The first thing to do is to start setting your bedtime and wake-up time at around the same time each day. Ideally, most people should get to sleep (not just in bed) before 11 p.m. to feel optimally rested and aim for around eight hours. If you are an exhausted warrior, you may need nine hours, whereas some scattered types may need less, e.g. seven hours.

The following are the parts of the sleep-reset protocol to start doing this week to help stimulate your body's natural sleep hormones, calm sleep-sabotaging stress hormones and reduce your brain's wakefulness areas in the evening to prepare for a deep restful sleep:

- Shut off all screens two hours before bedtime. Ideally, after dinner: no computers, smartphones or TVs past 7.30 p.m. for the next four weeks to really reset your sleep. After that, try to leave at least an hour before sleep of no screens, when you read a book, listen to music, meditate, have sex, relax with friends or do some gentle stretching or relaxing floor yoga poses. Scattered warriors have the most challenge with turning off screen time before bed, but it is one of the most important things to help them get to sleep and feel tired earlier so that they don't stay up until 2 a.m. on their phones.

- Change blue LED lightbulbs in your bedroom and living room to lower blue-light options: incandescent bulbs or blue-blocking light bulbs. This is especially important if you have trouble getting to sleep before midnight like many scattered warriors.
- Eat dinner by 7.30 p.m. latest. This is because late big meals can shoot up cortisol stress hormone at night and impair deep sleep cycles. If you get hungry later on, have a high tryptophan snack such as whole grain crackers with nut butter or cheese.
- Cut out all caffeine and alcohol for the next 4 weeks – wean down first if you are having more than 1 serving/day. Swap the alcohol for CBD mocktails and GABA-enhancing alcohol-free spirit to get the effect without the drama on sleep. Cutting the caffeine is most important for wound-up and exhausted types, while alcohol cutting out is important for all types.
- Lights out by 11 p.m. LATEST – sleep before midnight is better than sleep after midnight for most people, for all types, due to our clock genes. Of all the types, exhausted warriors may be most sensitive to needing this sleep before midnight.
- Avoid using your snooze button in the morning – if you must use an alarm, put the alarm on the opposite side of the room so you must get up to turn it off. Set your alarm for as late as possible instead of earlier with some 'snooze' alerts since the snooze time is not helpful for contributing to restorative sleep.
- Try to get bright light in the morning right after you wake up. This will help wake up your brain and also help set your body up to make more melatonin at night too. This is especially important for moody warriors.

If you are adding supplements this week:

- Order the supplements for everyone and consider the ones for your type, especially if your resilience score is in the below-50 range from taking the assessment in Part One. Start taking them this week to help get some 'quick wins'. There is a shortlist of supplements below. For the complete list of supplements for everyone and for your type, please refer to the supplements chapter in Part Two of this book for more detail. (Disclaimer: always check with your doctor or health practitioner before starting any supplements since a book cannot offer individualized advice. Some supplements may interact with other medications.)

For Everyone:
- High potency omega-3s: dose, for small fish sources 2–4g per day, or 1g per day for krill oil
- Magnesium biglycinate or glycinate: 400mg per day, in the evening
- Vitamin D oil drops dose range is between 1,000 and 5,000IU per day
- Full-spectrum CBD extract (cannabidiol) oil: dose varies but try starting with 5–10mg 2–3 times a day with a food for better absorption

For women under stress:
- Withania somnifera (ashwagandha/Indian ginseng): dose varies by product/extract, so check label

Additional specific supplements for your type:
Exhausted warriors
- Acetyl L-carnitine (another nutrient needed to help support mitochondrial function): 500mg three times a day
- Fat-soluble B-complex vitamin: 1–2 tablets per day

- Liposomal or S-acetyl Glutathione: generally the dose for fatigue and immune support is 600mg one to three times per day of liposomal, or 200mg per day and higher for the S-acetyl form
- Medicinal mushroom blend including cordyceps and reishi: for this supplement, it is important to choose a high-quality brand backed by a solid scientific formulation, since there is such a wide variation in the cheap versions versus more expensive brands in terms of potency and the amount of active plant compound content. The dosage will vary depending on the formulation

Wound-up warriors
- L-theanine: 200mg per dose, up to three times a day for anxiety, but start with once a day in the evening.
- Passionflower tablets or tincture taken in the evening: dose will vary by formulation/brand – see label on product.
- 50mg tryptophan: take an hour before bed.

Moody warriors
- SAM-e: stands for s-adenosylmethionine. The starting dose is around 400mg a day.
- Vitamin B12: to make SAM-e, you also need vitamin B12 so supplementing extra B12 even if your levels are in the 'normal' range may be helpful. Dose is 1 tablet per day.
- Saffron: dose generally is 15mg twice a day but may vary by product so check label.
- St Johns Wort: the dose is generally 300mg three times a day of a standardized extract product.

Scattered warriors
- For scattered warriors, it's all about supporting brain focus, concentration and memory.
- American ginseng dose will vary by product and formulation, check product label.

By the end of this week, you may be feeling more energized during the day and have less trouble falling asleep at night. Or, if a lot of these things were big changes, you may still be adjusting to temporary life without caffeine and alcohol and still not feeling great as your brain adjusts. That's OK too and totally normal. It can take four weeks or sometimes longer for long-held dysfunctional sleep habits to change and for the brain and body to adapt. Keep going with these changes and this programme for the next four weeks and I promise you will start to notice a change in the coming weeks. If this is taking up lots of mental bandwidth, stay with this week until you feel ready to move on to the week-two programme.

Week Two: Adding Resilience Resets and Turning on Your Relaxation Response

By this week, all or most of your supplements and CBD if you chose to start that have arrived, so organize them into your morning and afternoon stack and set a reminder to take them consistently.

This week is all about adding one-minute 'resilience resets' into your day, using a simple breathing practice and turning on your relaxation response, your inbuilt resilience helper which is the opposite of the fight-or-flight or stress response in the brain and body.

As the first step before we start activating our relaxation response, we have to identify your unique 'stress signature'. We will do this by doing a simple three-minute body scan practice (below) and writing down what you discover.

COMMON BODY SENSATIONS

- Tightness in shoulders, throat, chest, neck or jaw
- Lump in throat
- Funny feeling in stomach
- Dizziness, lightheadedness
- Sweating
- Feel heart beating fast
- Dry mouth
- Physical restlessness, feeling unable to sit still or needing to fidget, not able to stay comfortable sitting down while working (for example)

Here are some less physical signs of brain stress to watch for:
- Feeling anxious
- Mentally restless
- Frustrated
- Feeling overwhelmed
- Feeling brain-foggy
- Feeling low / impending dread
- Cravings for carbs, sugar or salt
- Feeling emotionally 'numb'

In addition to the above feelings and sensations that you may discover in your body-scan practice, you may also start to notice more general signs of stress throughout the day. So if you can't pin down a feeling or sensation but just get the general 'overwhelm' (wound-up warriors) or 'exhausted' (exhausted warriors) feeling, that's OK too: it can be part of your signature. Scattered types may just start to have more trouble focusing or staying organized. Once you start tuning in to what happens to you when you get stressed, you may also start to notice more specific signs like tight jaw muscles, or a repeated thought such as 'I can't cope' or negative self-talk, especially if you are a moody warrior, for example.

The Body-scan Instructions

Start by taking a few relaxed deep belly breaths and start bringing your attention back into your body and your breathing, noticing your belly and chest rise and fall. Don't try to change anything, just noticing without judgement. As you go, notice anything you feel, aches and pains, or tingling or thoughts or emotions that come up as you go. Don't try to change anything, just notice and explore. Then, starting at your feet, bring your attention gently to each part of your body: feet, shins, knees, thighs, pelvis, belly, ribcage and chest, up into your shoulders, then upper and lower arms, hands and fingers. Then bringing the attention back into your neck, up into the muscles of your face and head and then down your back, down the spine and over your back and towards the buttocks. When you finish the whole body, you can go back to any area you want to explore more, where you may have discovered stress or other sensations or feelings. Then gently bring your awareness back to your breath again. Notice any final thoughts or emotions as you breathe slowly in and out. End the practice with a few deep belly breaths and slowly open your eyes again.

WHEN TO DO IT

Throughout the day, check in with a one-minute body-scan practice after possible stress reaction triggers such as: after a cup of coffee or after a stressful moment at work. Write down in a note on your smartphone or in a paper journal you keep handy what body sensations, thoughts, emotions or feelings you can pick out that may be your brain's cue that it's stressed. To make sure you have enough chances to 'check in' on your stress signature, even if you don't notice any particularly stressful events today, set an alarm on your phone for a few scheduled check-ins throughout the day. Do you first check-in within thirty minutes of waking up, another check-in mid-morning around 10.30 a.m., another at lunchtime, one in the later afternoon around 4 p.m., and one around 9 p.m. as you start your sleep wind-down routine. Do this each day this week.

Now that you have identified your stress signature, you will be more aware of when and how stress starts to creep up on you during the day.

Next, using the simple breathing practice below, you can calm stress in the moment so it doesn't pile up, in as little as one minute. I call this one minute of breathing your 'resilience resets'. This is a practice for all types.

In addition to using the breathing practice for your one-minute resilience resets during the day to head off stress, start doing your breathing for five minutes as part of your pre-sleep routine in bed. This involves the belly breaths with a longer exhale, making that gentle *haaaa* sound as you breathe out, lying down with your eyes closed. This is especially important for wound-up warriors.

By the end of this week, you should be ending your day feeling less stressed, more energized and more in control of your stress levels. If you aren't there yet, don't worry, training your body and brain in the relaxation response does take time. If you are a wound-up warrior especially, this may take more time than for other types.

Also, remember to continue on the sleep-reset programme from last week.

Week Three (and Four): Resilience Diet

This week, it's time to take a look at your diet and how even small changes can make a big impact on your resilience by affecting your microbiome and changing how food affects things like your energy levels, stress-coping capacity and even things like your mood and mental clarity, depending on your type.

Making dietary changes involves cooking, planning and prep. I can tell you from experience as a busy working mum, that keeping on top of all of this is not always easy. Sometimes it means I buy relatively healthy prepared meals that use whole-foods ingredients I can just pop in the oven and throw them alongside some salad leaves or steamed veggies. That's the practical strategy I take with my patients too. The resilience diet is not about dietary perfection. If you can't cook and must resort to the best thing you can find in Pret a Manger, so be it! Eat your food slowly, mindfully and do a ten-second gratitude practice before you eat and you've instantly made that meal experience a healthier one.

So this week, start by looking at your current diet through a resilience diet lens and decide on between one and three changes you will make, based on the general resilience diet principles below. If it's 'cutting out refined sugar' or 'cutting out gluten', it may involve a kitchen-cupboard clean-out to put away, donate or remove those items for now.

You will notice some repetition in the foods list for each type if you already have read the full book including the diet chapter, but this is intentional to help give you a quick reference guide within this 8-week plan chapter.

- Eat at least two colours of vegetables at lunch and dinner, including cruciferous veggies (cauliflower, broccoli, Brussels sprouts), alliums (garlic, onions, shallots) or leafy greens such as mustard greens, kale and chard.
- Cut out added sugar in its many forms, including fructose, high-fructose corn syrup, glucose, etc. (This includes any form of

sugar added to processed or pre-made foods, snacks, granola, etc. – check ingredient labels.) Whole fruits and vegetables are allowed, even though they contain natural sugars.

- Reduce red meat intake to twice a week and change meats to grass-fed, organic and free-range.
- Eat one meal of small fatty wild fish (high in omega-3s) per week.
- Increase high-fibre foods. Sprinkle flax seeds on breakfast toast, yoghurt or muesli or in salads. Add in avocados, legumes (beans) and try an apple spread with nut butter for a snack.
- Cut out white carbs. This includes 'white' or 'wheat' bread, pastries, white pasta, white rice, pastries and normal pizzas, snack crackers, chips and cookies. Swap these for wholegrain varieties such as brown or wild rice, wholegrain 'sprouted' bread, wholewheat or brown rice pasta and wholegrain pizza bases (often in the frozen or fresh foods section) and healthier snacks like nuts and seeds, fruits, wholegrain baked crackers.
- Swap 'mixed vegetable oil' and low-quality pro-inflammatory oils with a combination of healthy oils.
- Cook with coconut or MCT oil.
- Increase MUFAs in oils such as cold-pressed rapeseed oil, olive oil and avocado oil to use on salads and in cooking and dips.
- Use organic butter and ghee.
- Have one serving of fermented foods per day. This can include using them in cooking. This includes kefir, yoghurt, kimchi, sauerkraut, tempeh (made from tofu) and miso, just to name a few.
- Cut out processed foods and sauces with ingredients that you cannot pronounce or with chemicals such as E-number dyes and food additives like carrageenan and synthetic low-calorie sweeteners, added flavour enhancers and MSG.
- Choose organic or unsprayed fruit and vegetables only, especially if eating the 'dirty dozen', i.e. the fruits and vegetables that are the most sprayed with pesticides. At the time of writing, these are: strawberries, spinach, kale, collard and mustard greens, nectarines, apples, grapes, bell and hot peppers, cherries, peaches, pears, celery and tomatoes.

- Cut out processed meats such as cold cuts, hot dogs, salami, deli meats, sausages.
- If you haven't already, cut out caffeine for the next four weeks.
- If you haven't already, cut out alcohol for the next four weeks.

These are some additional recommendations for food changes you may want to try based on your type.

WOUND-UP WARRIORS

Because calming a 'wound-up' nervous system is your challenge, you want to specifically support a calm balance via foods and drinks that contain building blocks to help make GABA, your body's calming brain chemical.

Increase/eat more of these:
- Fatty fish (i.e. wild salmon)
- Legumes
- Organic eggs from chickens and duck eggs
- Organic chicken
- Oats/oatmeal
- Yoghurt and kefir (organic, full fat and unsweetened, e.g. plain): to make them taste a bit nicer without adding sugar, you can add a dash of vanilla extract and/or liquid stevia
- Fermented soy products (i.e. tempeh, miso)
- Brown rice, quinoa, millet
- Tree nuts and seeds
- Water and herbal teas (mild dehydration causes an anxiety reaction in the body)
- Decaffeinated green tea (contains L-theanine for calming)
- Steamed (or raw) deep leafy greens with olive oil as a regular side dish at meals
- Salad greens
- Turkey
- Extra virgin olive oil for salads
- Cold-pressed coconut oil (for cooking)

- Specific foods high in taurine, which is an amino acid needed to make GABA: beef, lamb, dark chicken meat, eggs, dairy products, seaweed, krill and brewer's yeast (used for baking)
- Foods high in B6, which is the calming B vitamin great for wound-up warriors: chickpeas, beef and organ meats, potatoes, bananas, winter squash, nuts, non-citrus fruits

EXHAUSTED WARRIORS

Getting maximum energy out of your food and supporting mito-chondrial function is the main goal. Again, a diet high in refined, processed foods with chemical additives and preservatives may lead to worsening fatigue in many exhausted warriors, who tend to be extra-sensitive to these things. I have also found this resilience type does not generally do well on the 'all raw-food' diet and do better with at least some healthy cooked foods.

Dietary tips for your type: be aware of . . .
- Too much raw kale and raw cruciferous veggies: stick to cooked due to the possibility of these foods eaten raw being 'anti-thyroid' due to compounds in them called goitrogens. These compounds that can affect thyroid function may also worsen fatigue in some people.'For example, avoid putting raw kale in green smoothies and gently steam it instead.
- Any food you suspect you may have a sensitivity to (many exhausted warriors have hidden food intolerances, including foods that are high in histamine, or release histamine, lectins in some plant foods, or oxalates).
- *Increase foods high in N-acetyl cysteine or NAC, a glutathione precursor needed to make energy:* cruciferous vegetables are one of the richest food sources of glutathione, especially Brussels sprouts. Others include cauliflower, broccoli (particularly the flowers, not the stem), cabbage, kale, pak choi, cress, mustard, horseradish, turnips, swede. Just make sure they are gently steamed most of the time rather than raw.

- Garlic and shallots
- Avoid a totally raw diet
- Avoid (don't buy) any foods on the dirty dozen (page 247) completely unless you can get them organic/unsprayed.
- Minimize or cut out all wheat and gluten. Many exhausted warriors have an impaired gut barrier/gut lining or 'leaky gut' and tend to be sensitive to gluten, which can open the spaces in between the gut-lining cells and make leaky gut worse.

In addition to this, exhausted warriors may do very well on a 'keto-lite' diet, but have a hard time adapting to the dietary shift for the first two to four weeks. To test it out for yourself, ideally try to stick with it for six weeks and track your energy levels

If you have even a slightly sluggish thyroid, which can also cause fatigue, you may want to avoid excessive amounts of a few foods:

- Excessive amounts of raw cruciferous veggies such as raw kale as well as raw cabbage, cauliflower, and broccoli: gently steaming them first reduces the chemical that can interfere with thyroid function.
- Soybeans: genistein can be goitrogenic (i.e. it can cause thyroid goitres and thyroid problems in people who are prone to low thyroid or already have a thyroid problem if consumed in larger amounts, such as a main vegan protein source). Soy also is a high-pesticide crop, so organic only is recommended if you do eat a small amount.
- Millet: this grain in larger amounts can also be 'anti-thyroid', but in small quantities it is normally fine.

MOODY WARRIORS

For moody warriors, many find that their diet can have a huge impact on their moodiness. This is what I have found to be the best tips for your type:

- Eat mostly foods low on the glycaemic index: this is a blood-sugar-balancing diet and blood-sugar rollercoasters have a negative impact on mood and mood swings. If you google 'low glycaemic index foods', many free charts and infographics will pop up online, it's a long list.
- Consider going keto or keto-lite: keto diets have been used in small studies to treat depression and mood disorders and the associated fatigue that can often come with these conditions, as we touched on earlier.
- *Increase foods naturally high in folic acid: folic acid, or vitamin B9, is important for positive mood balance. The top foods for this are:*
  - Organic beef liver
  - Lentils
  - Asparagus
  - Avocados
  - Leafy greens (e.g. spinach)
  - Brussels sprouts
  - Beets
  - Walnuts
  - Flaxseeds
  - Citrus fruits (e.g. lemon, lime, grapefruit, oranges)
- *Increase Foods Rich in B12:*
  - Sardines, trout and salmon
  - Beef
  - Fortified nutritional yeast (this is a vegan-friendly source and can be added to many foods, marinades and salad dressings)
  - Organic milk and dairy products
  - Fortified mylks: these plant-based mylks do not naturally contain B12 so must have it added – check the label!
  - Vegan diets are low in B12 so generally supplements are recommended if you are strict vegan.
- *Increase foods high in tryptophan:*
  - Wild game meat, e.g. venison
  - Cottage cheese: goat's, sheep's or cow's

- White, kidney and soybeans
- Avocado
- Organic pork, duck, turkey and chicken meat
- Pumpkin seeds
- Wheat germ (only if you are not gluten intolerant; otherwise stick to the other items on this list)

SCATTERED WARRIORS

For scattered warriors, avoiding addictive cycles of food intake can be a challenge. Bingeing on 'moreish' foods can be an irresistible temptation. The cycle of food cravings and, in more extreme cases, food addiction has a brain basis. This craving cycle is worse with the more refined carbs and foods with a combination of high fat plus high carbs, such as potato crisps, desserts, junk foods and fried foods. So it's really important to minimize these if this is your type.

Many scattered warriors also find that intermittent fasting windows are helpful. This is where you try to eat your last meal earlier in the evening, e.g. by 6 p.m. and then not eat anything until breakfast at, say, 8 a.m. to give you a fourteen-hour 'fasting' window each day without skipping meals. Some scattered types actually do well with skipping breakfast to lengthen the fasting period, or eat the first meal at 10:30 or 11 a.m. instead of upon waking. Or try a 'bulletproof' high-fat coffee (black coffee blitzed with organic butter and/or coconut oil) as breakfast instead of foods and then eat the first meal around noon.

Scattered warriors should also increase their omega-3 fatty-acid-rich foods, especially from small coldwater fish or krill sources. Less bioavailable non-fish sources of omega-3s include hemp hearts, flax and chia seeds and walnuts.

After you have decided on the changes you will make, make a quick meal plan that considers your new eating habits. Try to pick two 'ready in ten minutes or less' recipes to make this week and buy ingredients. I also rely quite a bit on salads and high-fat meal smoothies with nut butters and yoghurt as the base in a pinch since these are more like three-minute meals for when you are extra busy. I recommend online grocery shopping and home delivery to let you plan things out in advance and cut the time spent going to the grocery store if that's an option for you.

This week, you may not notice a change in how you feel right away. In fact, when you change your diet to become healthier, you can actually feel worse for the first week and have cravings for the foods you cut out. That is normal and it will pass, generally around day seven, but possibly can take ten days if you have made some major shifts, such as cutting out refined carbs since they make up a huge percentage of the western diet.

Also remember that these changes take time and should be sustainable in the longer term, so it's better to make a small shift and stick to it than a huge change that is not sustainable. Food changes only work to help resilience and the microbiome as long as they are continued.

Week Four: Food Part Two

Continue with the changes you made last week. If you only made one small change and it went well and you want to add another one, go for it! Just make sure it's sustainable moving forward with both changes.

Check in with your sleep programme too: how are you sleeping now versus day one of week one? Are there any changes in how easy it is to fall asleep, waking up in the night, waking up less tired and total sleep time?

How are things going with your resilience resets to help decrease stress build-ups throughout the day? Are you finding you are able to notice your stress signature more easily now?

Celebrate any wins even if they seem small. They will continue to grow in the weeks to come!

Week Five: Developing Your Mind–body Practice

Congratulations! You are halfway through the resilience programme! The first part of the progamme focused on laying the groundwork for resilience with sleep, foods and supplements. It also got you doing your first minute mind–body practices with the body scan and the healing breath. This week, it's all about finding a more bespoke mind–body practice for your type to carry you forward and become a habit that will help boost your resilience and bust stress.

We will start with a future-self visualization. You can do this with a recording (there is a free one in our app* or you can search online) or using the detailed script in the mind–body chapter for self-visualization (page 199). Do this practice to start this week, ideally on a weekend or early evening where you have some time to listen to the recording or go through the script mentally for ten to fifteen minutes and then spend another few minutes reflecting on what came to you. This practice is a great way to get clear on why you are doing what you are doing in this programme, what you want out of your resilience programme and the way you want to feel as your best self. You may already feel like you are well on your way there after doing the first four weeks of this programme.

After you have done this practice, write down any personal insights you gained in a paper journal or on your smartphone or in the app. You can revisit this future-self practice once a season to renew it and see what's changed for you.

Next, choose a five-minute mind–body practice based on your type.

If you are having trouble deciding, start with mindfulness, which is beneficial to all types. For a detailed explanation of each practice, please see the mind–body chapter (page 181).

MOODY WARRIORS

- Loving-kindness or compassion meditations

---

* Free resources and recordings can be found at www.LondonResilience.com

- Gratitude practices such as Three Good Things and the Grateful Jar
- Activating moving meditation: Flying Goose
- Activating pranayamas (breathing) especially for the morning such as: bhastrika or kapalbhati, balancing breathing practices such as alternate nostril breathing (nadi shodhana)
- Altered states mind–body work through breath with guided holotropic breathwork, therapeutic psychedelics (where legal and appropriate for you: see the power plants chapter for details, page 159)

WOUND-UP WARRIORS

- For body noise (e.g. muscle tension in the face/neck or body, headaches), body-focused relaxation practices such as PMR (progressive muscular relaxation)
- For mind noise (e.g. not being able to shut off worried thinking, or mental chatter before sleep or rest): the Benson Technique
- Calming breaths such as the Healing Breath, Bee Breath

EXHAUSTED WARRIORS

- Yoga nidra recording practice: available online and in our app
- Mindfulness
- Energizing breath: bhastrika
- Cleansing breath: kapalbhati

SCATTERED WARRIORS

- Concentration meditation
- Mindfulness
- Focusing breath: ujjayi
- Balancing breath: nadi shodhana

After you have chosen your practice, pick a quiet spot at home where you will practise and set aside the same time each day if you can. Set an alert on your smartphone to remind you when to do it. It is really a personal choice when you do your short practice, but if you are not sure, try these tips for your type:

- Moody and scattered: try doing it as part of your pre-work morning wake-up routine
- Exhausted: at midday or mid-morning
- Wound-up: in the evening

At first, it may not feel like anything is happening but over the next six to eight weeks, the usual time it takes based on the mind–body research to see a significant brain effect, you will likely feel a significant shift in your resilience from this practice for just a few minutes a day. Most people find this becomes one of their favourite parts of their daily routine over time, once they get into a rhythm and over this initial learner phase of six to eight weeks.

Week Six: A Resilient Environment and Your Movement Practice

This week is all about two things: setting up a resilient environment and tuning in to your body's physical movement needs. Parts of this will look the same for everyone. Other aspects will be completely personal. So this week you'll need to really pay attention to your specific needs, rather than be guided entirely by the programme.

Environmental factors impact our resilience, from noise and light pollution to actual air pollution and chemicals in the foods we eat. This section could be an entire book on its own, but here we will touch on the most important aspects briefly this week for your home environment, since that is where we spend the most time and have the most control over things. You can start in just one room or area of your home at a time if it feels too overwhelming to do a whole house 'makeover' at once. Or you can also start with one category at a time, such as household cleaning products and swapping all or most for non- or lower toxicity options. (This is generally a great place to start, with a high return on investment!)

The process of learning about resilient environments can trigger anxiety and fear as we become aware of the multiple ways we are constantly exposed to environmental toxins in modern daily living. But I take comfort in the fact that even taking *any* steps to reduce your exposure and make your space healthier has a huge impact. It is actually impossible to avoid many or even most of these toxins completely because they are everywhere, so it's not about becoming obsessed, stressing or worrying if you can't afford fancy natural furniture or a hemp mattress, because stress is still the biggest toxin of them all. There are multiple studies showing that environmental toxins ranging from ingredients in plastics (including things such as Bisphenol A, or BPA, phthalates) as well as heavy metals, household chemicals and pesticides and fumes from paints and even home furnishings (called 'off-gassing') have negative effects on our brain, hormones and nervous system which can lead to problems managing stress, mood and energy issues as well as a risk of developing certain cancers.

The good news is that you can dramatically cut down the amounts of these chemicals you are exposed to and this is likely to have a really positive effect. For all things toxin-reducing, the Environmental Working Group or EWG website EWG.org is an excellent resource The focus here is not on creating an exhaustive list of chemicals you can't pronounce but to give you practical tips to put into practice this week.

Household Cleaning Products

Try to use more natural products, such as vinegar, baking soda and lemon juice mixed with some essential oils to make them smell nicer. This is what I use primarily, and where needed I occasionally buy 'eco-friendly' less toxic products such as toilet cleaners, etc. that contain less harmful chemicals and are often mainly based on apple cider vinegar and baking-soda mixtures. When shopping, products that have either a 'Green Seal' or 'Ecologo' certification are usually healthier options than those without these labels.

Indoor Air Quality

Since the start of the pandemic, indoor air quality has been brought to the forefront. In the last ten years, there have also been more research papers published that look at indoor air quality and the effects on health, from fumes from paint or building materials (which emit toxic substances called volatile organic compounds or VOCs) to cooking fumes, soft furnishings, mould and pollution from the street. Furniture, carpets and even mattresses, for example, are often coated with chemicals that prevent them from catching fire easily. These chemicals, called halogenated flame retardants or HFRs, are then released into the air in the process called 'off-gassing', especially when items are new.

WHAT YOU CAN DO

Because stress is also a major resilience buster, we don't want to create so much about perfecting your indoor air quality that it becomes all-consuming or creates anxiety (especially if you are a wound-up warrior like me!). However, the good news is that there are lots of things you can do to improve your indoor air quality, starting with some low-cost measures and working your way up the cost scale if you need to get more serious.

- *Lowest cost:* green up your space. Putting more plants inside the home is one of the best and cheapest ways to improve your air quality. Looking at plants also helps our mental health since our brains are soothed by nature, especially if you sit inside most of the day. You can also bring a plant to work for your desk or cubicle space and ask your workplace about considering more greenery to improve the office environment for better productivity and health. Some of the best indoor plant types for cleaning the air are:
  - Dieffenbachias
  - Peace lily
  - Golden pothos
  - Bamboo palms
  - Broad-leaved day palms
  - Variegated snake plants
  - Cornstalk dracaena
  - Weeping figs
  - English ivy
  - Devil's ivy
  - Philodendron
- Avoid burning things in the oven or toaster as much as possible. Burning things gives off fumes too, so when you do burn something (I am notorious for burning my sourdough toast in our house!), open the windows and turn on the extraction fan.
- As long as you are not right smack dab on a busy road with heavy traffic, open the windows to let the house breathe. When I used to live in central London, our front windows did unfortunately open right onto a busy traffic-choked road, so in the front of the house I actually kept the windows closed and used air purifiers instead and opened the back windows and doors.

- If you plan on painting, pay the extra for 'trace-VOC' paints. One company that we have used personally and that ships anywhere in the UK is called Graphenstone.
- Try to buy healthier furniture and mattresses when you are due to replace your current ones. This can be pricey, but look for second-hand to make it more affordable (that's what I do too). If you can't get around buying a new 'non-eco' furniture piece, let it air out for a few days if you can, either outdoors under a cover if possible or in a garage that is ventilated or with doors and windows open and/or an air purifier in the room to reduce the off-gassing fumes.
- Which brings me to the next one: air purifiers! There are so many to choose from and it's hard to know where to start. Generally speaking, the more expensive ones are better. However, for smaller rooms, you can get a decent-quality HEPA filter model for under a hundred pounds. The most important rooms to use it in are the bedroom (since you spend at least a third of the day sleeping in there!) and if you work from home, the home office or room where you work, especially if it's not well ventilated or near a window. This is something we have in the bedrooms and use overnight, especially in the damp cold winter months where the windows are open less.

Space Design and Set-ups

Removing clutter and leaving space is another free or nearly free (if you invest in some organizational kit) way to give yourself more mental headspace and reduce your mental stress load. This is especially important for scattered warriors, who tend to be the messiest type, although I certainly defy this generalization by being a very messy wound-up warrior! If the whole house seems too much to do, just try doing one room this week.

In addition to removing things and leaving more empty space, you can also think about adding a few elements such as aromatherapy natural candles or vaporizers: make sure you use the all-natural ones to avoid putting chemicals into the air.

Consider a change to lighting. Good lighting can completely transform the look and feel of space. Creating soft lighting, especially in spaces where you spend time in the evening, is important, and trying to avoid harsh fluorescent lightning wherever possible can help your brain wind down at night. If you are renting and can't overhaul the lighting fixtures (been there!), a floor lamp or two strategically placed table lamps are inexpensive and do the trick.

Finding Your Movement Practice

Movement is healing to the body and mind. It's also a way to get more feel-good brain chemicals and, best of all, it can be free. If you don't do any exercise or movement currently, just ten minutes of 'mindful' walking outdoors is a good way to start for all types. Mindful walking means walking without headphones or music or a podcast. Just be aware of your surroundings, the noises around you, the sights and any other physical sensations that bring you into the present moment.

Alternatively, to find your signature way to move, start by considering your resilience type. For example, wound-up warriors may find that calming movement practices like tai chi or hatha yoga work well for them. Exhausted types may find that walking and gentle stretching is a great fit to avoid overexertion from higher-intensity cardio exercise, especially when their reserves are low. Qi gong, a mind–body movement practice used to help with energy levels in traditional medicine may also help. For moody warriors, a brisk morning practice like jogging or a HIIT workout can help boost morning mood and motivation. For scattered warriors, a yoga practice that is more intense like ashtanga or one that requires concentration, like Iyengar, or a martial art can work well. However, if those feel uninspiring, you may need to choose something different. For example, incorporating dance in my home practice even for a few minutes a day is an important part of my movement routine, even on the days when I may go for a hike or jog outdoors. You may have to explore different movement practices or join a group to get a feel for a certain practice and see what suits you best. The most important thing is to move your body once a day in whatever way feels good, since movement is so important to both physical and mental wellbeing and ultimately resilience, no matter what your stage of fitness is.

So by the end of this week you should have made a few tweaks to your home and started to explore what your favoured way of movement is, something you can enjoy doing regularly in the long term to keep your body active and give you all the resilience benefits that any form of exercise brings. If you have tried a new exercise or movement form and it hasn't been a hit, don't despair. Keep exploring a new activity each month until you find your groove. I have patients who didn't find theirs until they were in their late fifties, when they finally took time to explore alternatives to the 'the gym' which they always hated. They took up curling, Nordic walking, Zumba and many other niche movement forms or types of yoga that finally made them feel excited about exercise rather than dreading it.

Week Seven: Passion and Spirit – Tuning In to What You Need to Thrive

This week is all about finding what brings more joy, connection, passion and purpose into your life. This may be slightly different depending on your type, but for all types it is about finding your passionate 'zest'.

Part of this passion/spirit week is also about reducing things that zap passion and 'zest'. One of the big ones is excessive screen time, which may change your brain's reward threshold, especially for scattered types. It can also cause more low moods, anxiety and zap energy (for moody, wound-up and exhausted warriors respectively). So this week, reduce 'browsing' time online and on social media. You can see in your phone settings how much time you spend in each app and social media in general each day to get an objective figure, which may surprise you!

Boosting Your Social Connectivity

Social connection is key to nurturing your spirit, no matter what your type, and being socially connected is one of the top ten resilience traits.

This week, aim for one point of contact with your social network each day by leaving a window of fifteen minutes to message or call a friend to say hi, grab coffee with a colleague you get on with or arrange a gym/workout/yoga class/walk with a friend or partner.

What works best can be different based on your type.

If you are a wound-up warrior, you may find that connecting in smaller groups or one-to-one works better than at big social events, which may feel overwhelming. If that's the case, plan a meet-up with one or a few friends this week for a walk, coffee or lunch. Talking through what is stressing you out with friends and having a laugh together is a proven way to lower your stress hormone levels and lower the overwhelm.

If you are an exhausted warrior and don't have much energy for connecting currently, think of some short, close-to-home catch-ups you can work into the week (meeting up with a friend who lives within a short walk for a coffee at your local, or having someone come to you for coffee/tea). When energy is at a real minimum, you can use voice messages on WhatsApp to stay in touch with friends and family if you don't feel up for an in-person or live video call catch-up. I use that strategy with my patients who suffer with chronic fatigue and need to work within their energy envelope so they don't get as isolated because of a lack of energy for 'live' meet-ups. If you are a moody warrior, when you go through a low patch it's a common habit to isolate further because of the fear of not 'being fun' or not being 'good company' or the worry about having to fake feeling happy. As scary as it can be, friends and family don't tend to judge our mood as we fear. If you are feeling low, consider picking an activity to do together that's more physical, like going to the gym, for a run or going to a yoga class together. Having the company will help get you out doing the thing you love and help you bust out of a low.

Blocking Out Your Me Time

This week, for all types, your other 'homework' is to find two blocks of one hour for passion discovery/me or fun time. Schedule these into your calendar, as well as your partner's/family's calendars if applicable, so everyone is aware you will not be available for duty at these two times. Think of these blocks as you would important work meetings so that they become 'high priority' and actually happen! If you don't know what to do with this time, here are some suggestions for your type:

SCATTERED WARRIORS

If you are a scattered warrior, tapping into your creativity, a natural superpower, takes you into your power zone and remind you of your many strengths. It doesn't have to be a traditionally creative hobby (but it certainly can be!). It's whatever you find that brings out your creative side, whether it's taking photos of your dog or creating some new music playlists to inspire different aspects of your day and week. Your homework this week is to find your creative outlet and do it in your two blocks of time. Then, moving forward, carve out at least one hour-long time block to keep it up each week.

WOUND-UP WARRIORS

Wound-up warriors tend to be overscheduled 'doers'. Your 'me time' this week may include something indulgent like going to get a massage or other spa treatment. Or reading a book and giving yourself permission to 'do nothing' or 'be lazy'. Or it may be going to do a candlelight evening-yoga or restorative-yoga class or watching a movie at home without being interrupted. If this is your type, you may feel guilty when you 'do less', but just know that this is a thought trap, not reality, and you are not only entitled to rest and relaxation, but you need it to balance your on-the-go nature.

MOODY WARRIORS

For moody types this week, it's extra important to give yourself a 'fun prescription', so you can have more 'Aha!' moments and break out of lows faster. Rediscover an old hobby that somehow got lost in the busyness of life or that you used to enjoy before a life change. For example, you may been a competitive athlete and when you quit the high level, you stopped doing it altogether. As hard as it can be to think of going back to something where you were at the elite level and are now only at a 'recreational' one, once you get over this fact it can bring you joy and connection just the same way as it used to, especially with team sports. Or, if that's not an option, try something altogether new that you've always wanted to do but have never got round to it. It could be something like a new sport or creative hobby which you know virtually nothing about but have an interest in. Consider taking a lesson in your chosen pursuit to try it out. Curiosity and not taking yourself too seriously are the names of the game.

The act of doing something new and different helps shake your brain out of stuck ruts, even if it doesn't turn out to be your new favourite hobby. The big thing with moody warriors is doing something – just taking action. You may feel that when your mood is low you don't enjoy doing things so it's better to do nothing. However, the act of doing something you have enjoyed in the past or trying something totally new helps kick the brain out of a low faster.

EXHAUSTED WARRIORS

When thinking of your 'me time', it's all about balancing your energy envelope (e.g. not using up more energy than you have in your tank) with the need to feel rejuvenated on a 'spirit' level. For example, you may absolutely love electronic music but going to a late-night music event leaves you too knackered to function. It could be finding earlier evening or even daytime event alternatives to get your music fix helps gets you excited again about this passion. You could also put together your perfect playlist at home and use Google to discover a new artist to add into the mix. Creative hobbies that don't require lots of physical energy can be a great fit too, from playing the piano to sketching, or taking photos with an old-school non-smartphone camera to avoid excess screen time. Or just sit outside in nature without any agenda.

Finding Your 'Aha!' Moments

You will start having more what are called 'Aha!' moments when you start reconnecting to your passions. 'Aha!' moments are moments and periods of dramatically enhanced mental clarity, calm focus and creative innovation. It's a special brain state when you are 'in your flow'.

Some passion activities that can trigger 'Aha!' moments, based on research from Harvard University, are listed on p. 230 in the mind–body chapter.

HOW TO GET STARTED

1. Write down your favourite things to do, hobbies, activities and passions/interests. Then add anything new you've been wanting to try but haven't yet. This can include activities but also things related to social connection like meeting a friend for coffee at your favourite local or watching a movie with a friend or partner.
2. Brainstorm how you can bring aspects of those interests or activities into your life again and schedule your 'me time' appointment into the calendar for two one-hour blocks this week and then one one-hour block after that (minimum) as a repeating

event in your virtual calendar.

By the end of this week, you should have started to tap into what brings you joy, makes you smile and connect more with your family and friends. You may have found that sharing your movement practice or the exercise routine you discovered in week six with a friend was the perfect way to get your social and movement fix in at the same time. Or that after you revamped the room in your house with less clutter and a few plants, you found the perfect space for a creative hobby.

Week Eight: Building Your Long-term Resilience Routine

After eight weeks (or longer if you turned each week into a phase of multiple weeks) of putting your resilience practices for your type into your life, you probably have an idea of what works best for you. What you have learned and put into practice over the course of this programme has helped you create what I like to call 'the resilient day'. This includes key habits at certain times of your day, like turning off screens at least an hour before sleep, as well as things to avoid based on your type.

Now is a good time to review how things have gone and create a stable daily routine moving forward that makes sense. Daily routines take time to build, and when you add something new, whether it's a new way of eating or even remembering to take magnesium before bed, it takes around two months to make it a habit. Once it reaches habit status, it starts to become a part of your day where you no longer need to use up significant mental energy to remind yourself to do it, like brushing your teeth. The key times to focus on for solidifying your resilience routines are in the morning, to help you start the day well, and in the evening, to help you unwind, calm your body and mind and prepare for rest and sleep. These are the two most important 'resilience' windows during the day to focus on and keep tweaking and checking-in on over time.

You can track the changes you have made and see your gains in your 'Resilience spectrum' score and the scores for your type over the past eight weeks in our free resilience clinic app. Tracking things can help you see what's changed the most, whether it's more energy, better mood, less stress or brainfog, or a combination of these things, so you can get really clear on what works best for you moving forward.

You may have found that you definitely feel better, for example, eating less sugar or avoiding caffeine and want to keep that going. Or you may find that after six weeks of no caffeine you haven't noticed any difference in your stress, anxiety, sleep and energy levels and you want to have a cup of coffee again to start the day.

On the mind–body front, you may have tried a meditation style for a few weeks and didn't gel with it so have moved on to another one that you have settled on now. If so, have you found a best time to set aside five minutes each day to practice? Is it in bed before going to sleep, or in the morning before breakfast? Or during your lunch hour? You can now set that as part of your daily routine.

Think about how you feel now. Do you feel overscheduled or overwhelmed, or are you ready to make even more resilience changes moving forward? What have you discovered about yourself in the past eight weeks in terms of likes and dislikes, challenges and superpowers? How can you use them to enhance your day moving forward?

Now is the time to review your progress and solidify in your daily routine the things you have been 'doing' and 'taking' that have made a difference in the way you feel so far. Now is also the time to make some decisions. For example, if you cut out alcohol and caffeine for a number of weeks and then introduced it back, did you notice a threshold for the amount of each of these you could consume without feeling poorly the next day? If even one or two drinks or cups of coffee made you feel worse after taking a 'holiday' from these substances, you might want to consider forming a new habit such as changing to Swiss Water decaf or only having a drink or two once a month. There are no rules, it's all based on your experiences.

By now, you probably have a good morning routine going, based on your regular waking-up time, what you eat for breakfast and any mind–body practice you may do in the morning before work. While your experiences are fresh in your mind, create a short ten-minute (weekday) and thirty minute (weekend) morning routine, chaining together key things from making breakfast, showering, personal care, etc. to whether you want to include a five-minute yoga or meditation practice to start the day off right, especially if the mornings are when you feel most motivated. This way, if you get into a rut in the future, which is totally normal, you have a quick guide to help get your mornings back on track.

Also be aware of resilience zappers as you move forward into the 'maintenance' phase of the programme and keep going with the positive changes you have made.

Physical resilience zappers include excessive screen time without taking mini breaks (one-minute resilience resets) during the workday, overconsuming 'energy-zapping' foods such as refined carbs and sugars, 'fake' sugars, processed foods with preservatives and also substances like caffeine, alcohol or other stimulants.

Mental resilience zappers will vary slightly based on your type. For wound-up warriors it's worrying and ruminating, for exhausted types it's people-pleasing or overcommitting, for moodys it's seeing things as glass half-empty, and for scattereds it's procrastination which leads to stressful rushing. So being aware of these traps if you find yourself in a rut in the future can help you bounce back faster once you recognize them as a classic for your type.

And lastly, when in doubt, under-schedule instead of overscheduling, make small changes and keep them going rather than a massive overhaul that can't last. It's also good practice for resilience to let our brains feel 'bored' occasionally, so don't worry about doing 'everything'. Sometimes 'doing nothing' is exactly what you need for your optimal resilience. So at least occasionally, embrace the experience of just being where you are, without feeling you need to keep improving or fixing things.

CONCLUSION

Your resilience journey is well under way by the time you read these words. I hope in these pages you have found inspiration, knowledge and comfort in knowing that resilience is your natural state of being and it's constantly evolving. It is never too late to change your resilience story. If you make even one small shift to tap into your resilience superpowers based on the recommendations for your type, whether it's taking a few minutes each day to just breathe and be kind to yourself or dipping your toes into the world of power plants, the rewards over time are exponential.

Even if you haven't yet made any of the recommended changes, but feel more compassionate and understanding towards yourself and your current challenges armed with the science of resilience, then this book has done its job. Maybe you learned something new about sleep and rest, or about how we actually need setbacks, challenges and stresses to grow our resilience, and that these are not intrinsically bad for us. There is no single path towards resilience, no right or wrong way to get there. Everyone's path is unique and finding your resilience type is simply a suggestion of where you may wish to begin.

If you've always been curious about meditation and how to discover your best-fit mind–body practice but never knew where to start, I hope that now you feel confident to explore and practice with curiosity and gentleness.

If you have always felt better eating certain foods or wondered why you like to skip breakfast but never knew why, or how to test what works best, you now have a starting point for how to use foods

273

as medicine and support your microbiome without going on a restrictive fad diet that can't last.

You may have had a cupboard filled with half-unused supplements because it's so confusing knowing where to start and what does what. I hope if you do choose to build your own resilience supplement stack, you now know where to confidently begin.

If you have been quietly curious about power plants but weren't sure who or how to ask, you can now understand these 'new medicines' free of past stigmas if you choose to explore using CBD yourself or using some of the more powerful tools in a guided, safe environment. You now possess the science behind them to allow you to be open minded and supportive to a friend or loved one who may find value in them instead of feeling frightened of their choice.

By making small changes at home, maybe you feel like you've been able to help your family feel more resilient too, by adding a few well-positioned plants around the house, using fewer chemicals for cleaning (my favourite excuse to clean less!) or consider getting a water filter (even though you still can't convince them to eat more greens). Sometimes resilience is about nurturing ourselves and our loved ones in whatever way feels best.

I hope that, whatever direction your resilience journey takes, you know that when things feel confusing, overwhelming or hopeless, you always have a resilience resource guide to come back to again and again to make your world a bit brighter, more joyful and figure-outable.

RESOURCES

For more resources on all things resilience, you can check out www.LondonResilience.com where you will find free resilience assessments and plans, guided meditations and our free app that lets you discover & test different resilience interventions to see what works best for you.

NOTES

Chapter 1: Finding Your Resilience Type

1   Weinberg, S.E., Sena, L.A. and Chandel, N.S., 'Mitochondria in the
     Regulation of Innate and Adaptive Immunity', *Immunity*, Vol. 42, Issue
     3, 2015, pp. 406–17.

2   Mills, E., Kelly, B. and O'Neill, L., 'Mitochondria are the powerhouses
     of immunity', *Nat Immunol* 18, 2017, 488–98.

3   West, A., Shadel, G. and Ghosh, S. 'Mitochondria in innate im-
     mune responses', *Nat Rev Immunol* 11, 2011, 389–402. https://doi.
     org/10.1038/nri2975

4   Myhrstad, M. C. W. et al., 'Healthy Nordic Diet Modulates the Ex-
     pression of Genes Related to Mitochondrial Function and Immune
     Response in Peripheral Blood Mononuclear Cells from Subjects
     with Metabolic Syndrome–A SYSDIET Sub-Study', *Mol. Nutr. Food
     Res.*, 2019, 63,1801405.

Chapter 2: The Science of Resilience

1   Rothman, M. and Mattson, M.P., 'Activity-dependent, stress-respon-
     sive BDNF signaling and the quest for optimal brain health and
     resilience throughout the lifespan', *Neuroscience*, Vol. 239, 2013,
     pp. 228–40.

2   Sinha, R. et al., 'Dynamic neural activity during stress signals resil-
     ient coping', *Proceedings of the National Academy of Sciences*,
     July 18, 2016, Vol. 113, Issue 31, pp. 8837–42.

3   Yirmiya, R. et al., 'Depression as a Microglial Disease', *Trends in Neu-
     rosciences*, Vol. 38, Issue 10, pp. 637–58.

4   Mecha, M., Carillo Salinas, F.J., Feliú, A. Mestre, L. and Guaza, C., 'Microglia activation states and cannabinoid system: Therapeutic implications', *Pharmacology & Therapeutics*, Vol. 166, 2016, pp. 40–55.

5   Kozłowska, U. et al., 'The DMT and Psilocin Treatment Changes CD11b+ Activated Microglia Immunological Phenotype', BioRxiv 2021.03.07.434103.

6   Slykerman, R.F. et al., 'Effect of Lactobacillus rhamnosus HN001 in Pregnancy on Postpartum Symptoms of Depression and Anxiety: A Randomised Double-blind Placebo-controlled Trial', *EBioMedicine*, Vol. 24, 2017, pp. 159–65.

7   Thorsell, A., and Mathé, A. A., 'Neuropeptide Y in Alcohol Addiction and Affective Disorders', *Frontiers in Endocrinology*, Vol. 8, 2017.

8   Li, T., Chen, X., Mascaro, J, Haroon, E. and James, K.R., 'Intranasal oxytocin, but not vasopressin, augments neural responses to toddlers in human fathers', *Hormones and Behavior*, Vol. 93, 2017, pp. 193–202.

9   Klimecki, O.M., Leiberg, S. Ricard, M. and Singer, T., 'Differential pattern of functional brain plasticity after compassion and empathy training', *Social Cognitive and Affective Neuroscience*, Vol. 9, Issue 6, June 2014, pp. 873–9.

10   Park, H. and Choi, E., 'Smartphone Addiction and Depression: The Mediating Effects of Self-esteem and Resilience among Middle School Students', *Journal of Korean Academy of Community Health Nursing*, Vol. 28, No. 3, Korean Academy of Community Health Nursing, pp. 280, 2017.

11   Arslan, G., 'Mediating role of the self–esteem and resilience in the association between social exclusion and life satisfaction among adolescents. Personality and Individual Differences', Vol. 151, 2019, 109514.

12   Kim, J. K. and Yoo, K. H. (2019), 'Effects of Self-esteem on Nursing Students' Resilience', *Journal of muscle and joint health*, 26(3), pp. 261–9.

13   Elvers P., Fischinger T., and Steffens J., 'Music listening as self-enhancement: Effects of empowering music on momentary explicit and implicit self-esteem', *Psychology of Music*, 2018, 46(3): 307–325. doi:10.1177/0305735617707354.

Chapter 3: The Circadian Rhythm Reset

1   Rijo-Ferreira, F., and Takahashi, J. S., 'Genomics of circadian rhythms in health and disease', *Genome Med*, 11, 82, 2019.

Chapter 4: The Resilience Diet

1   Zhang, C, Schilirò, T., Gea, M., Bianchi, S., Spinello, A., Magistrato, A., Gilardi, G., and Di Nardo, G., 'Molecular Basis for Endocrine Disruption by Pesticides Targeting Aromatase and Estrogen Receptor', *Int J Environ Res Public Health*, 2020, vol. 17, issue 16, 5664.

2   Aslam, H., Jacka, F.N., Marx, W., Karatzi, K., Mavrogianni, C., Karaglani, E., Mohebbi, M., Pasco, J.A., O'Neil, A., Berk, M., Nomikos, T., Kanellakis, S., Androutsos, O., Manios, Y., and Moschonis, G., 'The Associations between Dairy Product Consumption and Biomarkers of Inflammation, Adipocytokines, and Oxidative Stress in Children: A Cross-Sectional Study', Nutrients, 2020, vol. 12, issue 10, 3055.

3   Labonté, M-È., Cyr, A., Abdullah, M.M., Lépine, M-C., Vohl, M-C., Jones, P., Couture, P. and Lamarche, B., 'Dairy Product Consumption Has No Impact on Biomarkers of Inflammation among Men and Women with Low-Grade Systemic Inflammation', *The Journal of Nutrition*, vol. 144, issue 11, November 2014, pp. 1760–1767.

4   Camfield, D., Owen, L., Scholey, A., Pipingas, A., and Stough, C., 'Dairy constituents and neurocognitive health in ageing', *British Journal of Nutrition*, 2011, vol. 106, issue 2, pp. 159–174.

5   Melnik, B.C. and Schmitz, G., 'Pasteurized non-fermented cow's milk but not fermented milk is a promoter of mTORC1-driven aging and increased mortality', *Ageing Research Reviews*, 2021, Volume 67.

6   Neth, B.J., Mintz, A., Whitlow, C., Jung, Y., Sai, K.S., Register, T.C., Kellar, D., Lockhart, S.N., Hoscheidt, S., Maldjian, J., Heslegrave, A.J., Blennow, K., Cunnane, S.C., Castellano, C-A., Zetternerg, H. and Craft, S., 'Modified ketogenic diet is associated with improved cerebrospinal fluid biomarker profile, cerebral perfusion, and cerebral ketone body uptake in older adults at risk for Alzheimer's disease: a pilot study', *Neurobiology of Aging*, Volume 86,v 2020, pp. 54–63.

7   Paoli, A., Mancin, L., Giacona, M.C. et al., 'Effects of a ketogenic diet in overweight women with polycystic ovary syndrome', *J Transl Med*, 2020, vol. 18, issue 104.

8   Alwahab, U.A., Pantalone, K.M., and Burguera, B., 'A Ketogenic Diet may Restore Fertility in Women with Polycystic Ovary Syndrome: A Case Series', *AACE Clinical Case Reports*, vol. 4, issue 5, 2018, pp. e427–e431.

9   Michalczyk, M.M., Klonek, G., Maszczyk, A., and Zajac, A., 'The Effects of a Low Calorie Ketogenic Diet on Glycaemic Control Variables in Hyperinsulinemic Overweight/Obese Females', *Nutrients*, 2020, vol. 12, issue 6: 1854.

10   Heilbronn, L.K., Civitarese, A.E., Bogacka, I., Smith, S.R., Hulver, M., and Ravussin, E., 'Glucose tolerance and skeletal muscle gene expression in response to alternate day fasting', *Obesity Research*, 2005, 13(3), 574–581. https://doi.org/10.1038/oby.2005.61

11   Leung, M.C.K. and Meyer, J.N., 'Mitochondria as a target of organophosphate and carbamate pesticides: Revisiting common mechanisms of action with new approach methodologies', *Reproductive Toxicology*, Vol. 89, 2019, pp. 83–92.

Chapter 5: Resilience Supplements

1   Reddy, P. and Edwards, L.R., 'Magnesium Supplementation in Vitamin D Deficiency', *American Journal of Therapeutics*, Vol. 26, Issue 1, January/February 2019. pp. e124–e132.

2   Barbagallo, M., Veronese, N., and Dominguez, L. J., 'Magnesium in Aging, Health and Diseases', *Nutrients*, 2021, 13(2):463.

3   Shen, Y., Dai, L., Tian, H., et al., 'Treatment Of Magnesium-L-Threonate Elevates The Magnesium Level In The Cerebrospinal Fluid And Attenuates Motor Deficits And Dopamine Neuron Loss In A Mouse Model Of Parkinson's disease', *Neuropsychiatr Dis Treat.*, 2019;15:3143-3153. Published 2019 Nov. 11. doi:10.2147/NDT.S230688.

4   Laird, E., Rhodes, J. and Kenny, R.A., 'Vitamin D and Inflammation: Potential Implications for Severity of Covid-19', *Irish medical journal*, 2020, 113, 81.

5   Abboud, M., Rizk, R., AlAnouti, F., Papandreou, D., Haidar, S., and Mahboub, N., 'The Health Effects of Vitamin D and Probiotic Co-Supplementation: A Systematic Review of Randomized Controlled Trials', *Nutrients*, 2021, 13(1):111.

6   Amirani, E. et al., 'The effects of probiotic supplementation on mental health, biomarkers of inflammation and oxidative stress in patients with psychiatric disorders: A systematic review and meta-analysis of randomized controlled trials', *Complementary Therapies in Medicine*, Vol. 49, 2020, 102361.

7   Yu, J., Cao, G., Yuan, S. et al., 'Probiotic supplements and bone health in postmenopausal women: a meta-analysis of randomised controlled trials', BMJ Open, 2021, 11:e041393.

Chapter 6: The Power Plants for Resilience

1   Yang, Y., Maher, D.P. and Cohen, S.P, 'Emerging concepts on the use of ketamine for chronic pain', *Expert Review of Clinical Pharmacology*, 13:2, 2020, pp. 135–146.

2   Dore, J. et al. 'Ketamine Assisted Psychotherapy (KAP): Patient Demographics, Clinical Data and Outcomes in Three Large Practices Administering Ketamine with Psychotherapy', *Journal of Psychoactive Drugs*, 51:2, 2019, pp. 189–98.

3   Maudlin, B., Gibson, S. B., and Aggarwal, A., *Intern Med J.*, published online 6 June 2021.

Chapter 7: Mind–body Resilience

1   McEwen, B., 'In pursuit of resilience: stress, epigenetics, and brain plasticity', *Ann. N.Y. Acad. Sci.*, 1373, 2016, 56–64.

2   Moszeik, E.N., von Oertzen, T. and Renner, K.H., 'Effectiveness of a short Yoga Nidra meditation on stress, sleep, and well-being in a large and diverse sample', *Curr Psychol*, 2020.

3   Ferioli, M., Zauli, G., Maiorano, P., Milani, D., Mirandola, P., and Neri, L. M., 'Role of physical exercise in the regulation of epigenetic mechanisms in inflammation, cancer, neurodegenerative diseases, and aging process', *J Cell Physiol.*, 2019; 234: 14852–64.

4   Takakura, S., Oka, T., and Sudo, N., 'Changes in circulating microRNA after recumbent isometric yoga practice by patients with myalgic encephalomyelitis/chronic fatigue syndrome: an explorative pilot study', *Biopsychosoc Med.*, 2019 Dec 2; 13:29.

ACKNOWLEDGEMENTS

As ever, this work and this book would not be possible without my patients and clients who bravely share their stories and resilience journeys with me and allow me to be a part of their healing.

To my husband and resilience partner in crime, Nick, for always encouraging and supporting me and going on many crazy adventures together over the years in search of new ways to become more resilient. To my son River, my little resilience teacher who brings a smile to my face and puts everything into perspective even on the most stressful of days, you light up my life. And thanks to my wonderful family, my mum and mum-in-law Chris for their support, love and open-mindedness to all the slightly unconventional things I do in the name of resilience both personally and professionally!

I am also so grateful for my wonderful integrative and cannabinoid medicine colleagues around the world, who I am constantly learning from.

Thank you to my incredible agent Rachel Mills, Alexandra Cliff and their amazing team at RML, and my UK editing guru Pippa Wright and her team at Orion Spring for being the dream team to work with and supporting this book with so much love.

ABOUT THE AUTHOR

Dr Dani Gordon is a double board certified medical doctor, writer, speaker and world-leading expert in integrative and cannabinoid medicine. She is the founder of The London Resilience Clinic, a leading medical clinic specialising in fatigue, mental health and pain conditions and LondonResilience.com a platform offering personalised holistic resilience programs to help people bounce back better. After completing her family medicine residency at the University of British Columbia in Vancouver, she went on to become an American board qualified specialist in integrative medicine and now practices in the UK. She is the Vice Chair of the UK Medical Cannabis Clinician Society and a policy advisor the Conservative Drug Policy Reform Group. She has been featured in numerous TV and media publications including *Vogue*, *Forbes*, *The Sunday Times*, *The Guardian*, BBC and Channel 4.

She lives in Buckinghamshire with her husband Nick, her son River and Indica (Indy) the cavapoo.

Orion Credits

Orion Spring would like to thank everyone at Orion who worked on the publication of *The Resilience Blueprint*.

Agent
Rachel Mills

Copy-editor
Sarah Hulbert

Editor
Pippa Wright

Proofreader
Francine Brody

Editorial Management
Clarissa Sutherland
Frances Rooney
Carina Bryan
Jane Hughes
Charlie Panayiotou
Tamara Morriss
Claire Boyle

Audio
Paul Stark
Jake Alderson
Georgina Cutler

Contracts
Anne Goddard
Ellie Bowker

Design
Nick Shah
Jessica Hart
Joanna Ridley
Helen Ewing

Picture Research
Natalie Dawkins

Finance
Nick Gibson
Jasdip Nandra
Sue Baker
Tom Costello

Inventory
Jo Jacobs
Dan Stevens

Marketing
Helena Fouracre

Production
Katie Horrocks

Publicity
Frankie Banks
Ellen Turner

Sales
Jen Wilson
Victoria Laws
Esther Waters
Group Sales teams across Digital, Field Sales, International and Non-Trade

Operations
Group Sales Operations team

Rights
Rebecca Folland
Barney Duly
Ruth Blakemore
Flora McMichael
Ayesha Kinley
Marie Henckel

INDEX